# Theory and Methods in Dance-Movement Therapy

THIRD EDITION

Penny Lewis Bernstein Ph.D.
Registered Dance Therapist
Antioch University
Antioch-New England Graduate School
Keene, New Hampshire

AF859586

KENDALL/HUNT PUBLISHING COMPANY
Dubuque, Iowa, USA • Toronto, Ontario, Canada

Copyright © 1972, 1975 by Penny Lewis Bernstein

Copyright © 1981 by Kendall/Hunt Publishing Company

ISBN 0–8403–2378–6

All rights reserved. No part of this publication may be reproduced, stored in a retrieval system, or transmitted, in any form or by any means, electronic, mechanical, photocopying, recording, or otherwise, without the prior written permission of the copyright owner.

Printed in the United States of America B 402378 01

*about the cover . . . . .*

*The spiral mandala of wo/man's experience of being-in-the-world ebbs and flows like the tide with the Self as the central axis of the vortex.*

*Within each person lies the sum total of his life from pre-birth to the present. When fully integrated, adaptive developmental schemata can provide the foundation and direction for the evolving personal journey.*

*P.L.B.*

To Lynne, Ann, Judy, and Irma

# CONTENTS

Appendix

# PREFACE

It cannot be emphasized enough that this book is not in any way a "cook book." "Cook books" in the field of human behavior do gross injustice to the subject matter as well as to everyone involved. Examples are given of ways of looking at maladaptive behavior and treatment. They are as stated: examples—certain possibilities among many. It is hoped also that all elements discussed will be seen within the context of the sequence of the characteristic movement repertoire of the client and as they relate to the total human being and his way of life.

Each individual has his own timing as to his readiness for exploring a certain aspect of his psychology. Although the therapist may know instantly from observing his body movement repetoire that he has not sufficiently integrated certain parts of his being, it is the client/patient who consciously or unconsciously dictates the area and depth of the therapeutic engagement. Suggestions by the therapist for movement explorations need to flow from the client/patient's own process with the same ease by which one drop in a stream of water is wedded to another.

The theoretical frame of reference was selected because of its applicability and relevance with existing data in this field as well as its success in other areas of mental health and neurophysiologic rehabilitation. The theory utilized is that of the recapitulation of ontogeny, i.e., the recreation of the basic elements in life which are thought to be responsible for normal development. The theory is based on the premise that an individual who has difficulty functioning adequately will be able to live more successfully by organizing and integrating those components of psycho-motor maturation which are usually experienced in the normal growth process. Dance-Movement Therapy is seen as a process entailing the use of developmentally oriented body movement for awareness, expression, exploration, identification, and integration toward an experience of wholeness.

Because of its developmental base, this book should be useful not only to the dance therapist, but also to individuals who are involved with the primary prevention of psychomotor pathology—the physical educator, movement specialist, occupational therapist, and physical therapist—and those mental health professionals who are seeking a more holistic approach to their work with individuals.

# ACKNOWLEDGMENTS

Without the many hours spent by Dr. Judith Kestenberg going over and reinforcing her way of evaluating and looking at development through movement, much of this book would have suffered. Thank you, Judy.

I am also indebted to Irmgard Bartenieff who contributed much time and effort in reading and discussing the conceptual and experiential aspects of the book.

And finally, to my clients and students who have taught and continue to teach me what no book or course could ever begin to, thank you all.

P.L.B.

# CHAPTER I

# Dance-Movement Therapy: Its Rationale and the Development of a Theoretical Frame of Reference

## MIND-BODY GESTALT

Duality is an illusion. The salience of this premise has particular relevance to recent rediscoveries in the relationship between mind and body. The holistic view of the individual, acknowledging the complex interrelationship between psyche and soma, is becoming operationally acknowledged. The line between what is a "purely physical illness" and an "emotional problem" has been dissolving. Even the predisposition of individuals for placing themselves in harm's way for traumatic accidents is not out of the range of psychosomatic determinants. It was Freud who first conceptualized the mind-body entity. He stated, "Emotions and instinctual gratifications and feelings of frustrations do not consist of mere thoughts but of physical alterations."[1]

## NATURAL FLOW OF ENERGY

These so-called alterations occur through the transmission of psychic energy to certain related muscles, organs, and/or physiological processes. In an adaptive, functioning individual, as in all life forms, there occurs a natural flow of energy. This flow can be altered by internal conflict and the lack of an integrated experience of wholeness. The keys to understanding the rationale behind why individuals hold their muscles and thus their bodies in particular postures, why breathing is executed in various manners, why certain people are prone to accidents, and why illnesses effect particular physiologic organ systems all lie in personal psychosomatic histories.

## SEQUENTIAL DEVELOPMENT

As with all other life forms, a human being develops in an organized sequential manner. Each phase of development has its somatic, physiologic, and psycho-social elements, all of which are interrelated and necessary for the

1. Felix Deutsch, M.D., *On the Mysterious Leap from the Mind to the Body.* (New York: International University Press, 1973) p. 7.

resolution and organization of each ontogenic phase. If individuals do not have the appropriate internal and external environment to develop, phase-related maladaptive experiences get stored in the body. The specific muscular system or physiological organ in which these experiences are cathected depends on their primacy or symbolic relationship to a person's development. Thus an individual may be autistic or psychotic, or may have chronic tension, habitual behavioral patterns, ulcers, asthma, low back pain, cystitus, continual injuries to one or more limbs, or even cancer in a specific organ—all of which may be due to inadequate development in particular phases.

## USE OF DANCE-MOVEMENT THERAPY

Dance-movement therapy has its roots in the shamanistic tradition in which the roles of priest, medicine man, and emotional healer were all executed by one person. The shaman's healing powers were often carried out with movement. Meerloo writes, "The dance of the medicine man, priest, or shaman belongs to the oldest form of medicine and psychotherapy in which the common exhaltation and release of tensions were able to change man's physical and mental suffering into a new option on health."[2]

For some time, human beings have lived in an era of specialization. If a person has eczema, he goes to a skin doctor; for chronically tense muscles and joints he sees an orthopedic person or chiropractor; with acute depression one engages a psychiatrist. Quite often symptoms are treated without so much as a thought regarding their etiology. Even in depth psychoanalysis the physical symptom is not directly dealt with, but rather is expected to dissipate with the success of the "talking cure."

The movement therapist, on the other hand, not only acknowledges the mind-body gestalt, but is one of the few healing professionals who engages the individual from both foci. Breathing patterns, body attitudes, and movements, as well as the organ systems, are dealt with simultaneously with the individual's conscious and unconscious verbal expressions.

The use of body movement as a tool in the therapeutic process is perhaps even more relevant today in our highly "civilized" culture than it has been in so-called primitive cultures. Movement can provide a direct, unedited avenue into the developmentally based origins of psycho-physiologic maladaptions. Based on recent research, Israel Zwerling, M.D., remarks about movement therapy that it "evokes responses precisely at the level at which psychotherapists seek to engage their patients more directly and immediately than do

2. Joost A. Meerloo, *Creativity and Eternalization.* (New York: Humanities Press, 1968) p. 69.

the more traditional verbal therapies."[3] It is the unconscious which has, since Freud, been considered the storehouse for repressed conflict, unintegrated experiences, and painful psycho-social traumata.

Free associational, authentic movement from the primary process world of the unconscious provides not only images and verbal reflections, but it can totally engage the person in re-experiencing the developmentally based environments which negatively influenced his natural development. These same types of movement experiences can allow the individual to explore the elements required for building strong foundations.

Another factor concerning the use of movement is the acknowledgment of the primacy of body movement in communication. It is through the often subtle nuances of mothers' movements that infants first learn to trust or mistrust their environment and to feel positively or negatively about themselves. And it is through the use of empathetic movement reflection by the dance therapist, that the most severely disturbed psychotic, autistic, or organically disabled can begin to be engaged in a therapeutic object relationship which will gradually provide the needed elements for healthy development.

Finally, dance-movement has been employed in many cultures since the inception of civilization as a vehicle through which communities assist individuals through life's rites of passage and as a means through which persons relate to the forces which govern their survival.[4] Much of this dancing involves repetitive rhythmic body action. Through communal expression, participants have often experienced personal transformations. Ecstasy and transpersonal relatedness are not uncommon phenomena in this type of group dance.[5]

With hospitalized individuals whose affectual expressions have been atrophied due to continuous pervasive maladaptive environments, group rhythmic dance can afford the needed conduit through which they can begin to risk moving from their unconscious psychotic world into the conscious world of relatedness.

The capacity of rhythmic body action to provide a bridge between the conscious and unconscious world makes it a powerful tool with all populations. Those who need a way back into consciousness and those who need to explore a way into the world of symbolic expression can all benefit. The group can afford the participant a powerful reverberation and organization of needed developmentally related aspects of their psychology.

3. Israel Zwerling, "The Creative Arts Therapists: Struggling for Recognition." *Hospital and Community Psychiatry,* Vol. 30, No. 12, Dec., 1979, p. 843.

4. Bernstein, Penny, *Eight Theoretical Approaches in Dance-Movement Therapy.* (Dubuque: Kendall/Hunt Pub, 1979).

5. Bernstein, Penny, & Leah Hall, "Cross-Cultural Puberty Rituals and Jungian Dance Therapy: A Comparative Study." Paper presented at the First International Dance Therapy Association Conference, Toronto, 1977.

## IDENTIFICATION AND DEFINITION OF CONCEPTS AND HYPOTHESES WHICH DIRECTLY APPLY TO THE THEORY OF RECAPITULATION OF ONTOGENY IN DANCE-MOVEMENT THERAPY

### Concepts

*Dance-Movement Therapy*—is a process entailing the use of developmentally based body movement for awareness, expression, identification, exploration and integration toward the experience of wholeness.[6]

*Adaptive Patterns*—are those integrated components of an individual's psychology which enable the capacity to meet self needs and fully experience being-in-the-world.[7]

*Developmental Task*—is the process of learning in an integrated manner a developmentally based adaptive pattern.

*Maladaptive Behavior*—is behavior which either does not adequately serve toward the satisfaction of self needs or demonstrates an inability to fully experience being-in-the-world.

*State of Function*—An individual may be said to be in a state of function when he has organized in an integrated manner those adaptive patterns which are in service toward the satisfaction of self needs and toward the capacity to fully experience being-in-the-world.

*State of Dysfunction*—An individual may be said to be in a state of dysfunction when he has not fully organized in an integrated manner those adaptive patterns which are required in order to satisfy self needs and fully experience being-in-the-world.

### Hypotheses

*Process of identifying the function-dysfunction continuum*—The individual's state of function or dysfunction may be assessed through the observation of his somatic behavior. Either component-related maladaptive behavior or behavior which exhibits adaptive components may be observed while the individual is participating in total movement activities requiring the use of adaptive patterns.

Verbal associations to past, present, and future life experience may serve to enrich the identification process.

*Movement from a State of Dysfunction to Function*—This is a therapeutic process which occurs though engagement in and integration of developmentally based intra and interpersonal movement, verbal associations to the unconscious along with connections to past, present, and future life experience.

6. Penny Bernstein, Ed., *Eight Theoretical Approaches in Dance-Movement Therapy* (Dubuque: Kendall/Hunt Pub., 1979).

7. Some concepts, hypotheses, and theory have been adapted from Anne Mosey, *Occupational Therapy: Theory and Practice* (Medford: Pothier Bros. Printers, 1968).

## Summary

The theory of recapitulation of ontogeny states that any individual who has difficulty in functioning adequately in body movement will be able to live more successfully by organizing those adaptive patterns which are usually integrated in normal development. The organizing process may occur in total movement activities which incorporate the components usually acquired in normal human development. The specific patterns utilized depend upon the most basic level at which the individual is able to function. Through various movement-based experiences using higher complexities of developmental tasks, the therapist assists the individual in evolving to his age-appropriate level of functioning.

Within this framework, the therapist keeps in mind what is idiosyncratically and socio-culturally adaptive for each individual such that the desired movement repertoire is a natural expression for the individual within his environment.

## Further Consideration and Application

This theory is easily adaptable to almost any approach utilized in psychotherapy whether it be an intensive care psychoanalytic sanatorium, outpatient community mental health center, special education facility, holistic health clinic, or private practice. Although the foundations are in neurophysiology and psychotherapy, the theory stresses the practical organizing of abilities which are needed in everyday life. Further flexibility is built in the realization that not all individuals need to organize all the adaptive patterns which will be recorded in the following chapter. Treatment plans will be influenced by, among other things, the client's chronological and mental age, his previous cultural socialization, and the socio-economic environment to which he returns.

It should also be noted that although these patterns are sequential, the patient himself determines by his actions and abilities the degree of emphasis placed at each level. Equal time is not always given to each adaptive pattern. This is particularly true when treatment is directed toward a regressed individual who has already partially organized many of the areas. Once early levels, i.e., the foundation, are in place, the recapitulation process may progress toward the appropriate level of development at a quicker pace. The end goal and progress for each individual is therefore specifically related to his own needs and rhythmic patterns of growth.

This theory is not based on the usual nomenclature of medical diagnosis; however, for reasons of familiarity and clarity, the standard classifications will be employed. By definition it would seem that those who are in a state of dysfunction had never integrated or organized the patterns or had attempted to learn them but, due to inadequate integration of a foundation level, were somewhat impeded and ineffectual in functioning at higher and more complex levels. Autistic children, as well as individuals suffering from schizophrenia, seem especially to fall into one of these categories; however, various disorders[8] such as infancy, childhood and adolescent disorders particularly those of the developmental, movement, and/or emotional categories, are also highly appropriate. Somatoform disorders with psychosomatic and psychophysiologic symptomatology are directly applicable.[9] Psychosexual and affectual disorders are also well suited to this form of therapy.[10] Those diagnosed with personality disorders, typically difficult to treat, have been able to develop working alliances with therapists who allow for the potential for sensori-motor object relationship. Borderline and narcissistic personalities have both benefited from a developmental movement therapy approach.[11, 12]

Although this theory is specifically designed for the treatment of those in a state of emotional dysfunction by dance-movement therapists, there are other areas of rehabilitation and/or growth which might benefit from its utilization. For example, use of this theory may be made in attempting to "re-adapt" culturally deprived children to the types of abilities needed for adequate functioning in a society which stresses other adaptive patterns.

Students in a normal school setting could also benefit from a teacher who is knowledgeable in the underlying age-specific body-movement patterns needed by individuals in order to function adequately. By being able to detect at what level the difficulty in the organization of a behavior or skill becomes apparent, elementary classroom teachers and physical education teachers could be better able to instruct and evolve their students to higher levels of ability and adaptability in psycho-motor organization and integration.

8. *Diagnostic and Statistical Manual of Mental Disorders—DSM-III* (Washington, D.C.: American Psychiatric Assoc., 1980).

9. Bernstein, Penny, "A Mythologic Quest: Jungian Movement Therapy with the Psychomatic Client," *American Journal of Dance Therapy*, vol. 3, no. 2, 1980.

10. *Ibid.*

11. Seigel, Elaine, "Psychoanalytically Oriented Dance-Movement Therapy—A Treatment Approach to the Whole Person" *Eight Theoretical Approaches in Dance-Movement Therapy, op. cit.*

12. Author's clinical experience and discussions with other movement therapists.

# CHAPTER II

# The Learning Process

The learning of adaptive patterns is supported by two related concepts in the theory of development: (1) Werner's principles of orthogenesis and (2) Piaget's process of equilibration.

Orthogenesis may be defined as follows:

1. increasing differentiation and specification of primitive action systems causing
2. the emergence of novel discrete action systems that are also increasingly integrated within themselves.
3. The most advanced systems functionally subordinate and regulate less developed systems.[1]

This definition generally states that in the course of normal development action systems become more and more complex and differentiated.

Equilibration, on the other hand, is "a process of 'formative instability combined with progressive movement toward stability.' Its course is spiral and consists of 'progressive involutions by which structure and function are jointly matured.' "[2]

When these two concepts are combined, learning can be seen as an active process whereby more and more complex action systems are differentiated and specified causing progressive states of disequilibrium which result, through the need to re-obtain equilibrium, in more complex novel discrete action systems.

Thus, a spiral process of development may be visualized, with each new level of complexity growing out of the last.

Like most developmental theorists, Piaget feels that normal growth is not solely a physiological experience; it is rather an interactional process between the environment and the individual. If the environment does not supply the appropriate elements for the learning and integrating of more organized levels, the transition to the next level will be inadequate.

1. Jonas Langer, *Theories of Development* (New York: Holt, Rinehart and Winston, 1969), p. 92.
2. *Ibid.*, p. 93.

Therefore, in order for the learning of a particular level in functioning to take place, the individual must not only have arrived at a sufficient maturational level, have fully organized all the past—and less complex—levels of functioning, and have progressed into a state of disequilibrium; but he must also be in an adequate and appropriate environment which has all the necessary elements in order for learning to occur.

The environment can be seen as either representational and/or symbolic of the appropriate environment needed to fully integrate a higher level of functioning. Therapy has its own ritual process which resembles its shamanistic forbearers. The client/patient disidentifies from more primitive levels of functioning through the development of a therapeutic object relationship and the provision of an environment for the re-experiencing of existant maladaptive patterns (disequilibration). As their origins are clarified, these patterns are gradually replaced by more age appropriate adaptivity. This therapeutic rite of passage results in a new, more complex re-integration and an expanded experience of the self (re-equilibration). This may occur through the client's engagement in unconscious free associational active imagination authentic movement; or it may entail a transferential movement interaction between client/patient and therapist; or it may involve group rhythmic interaction with specific props and music.

# CHAPTER III

# Developmental Constellation

The following 16 areas of organization will give the reader an idea of the various ways of looking at ontogeny and the corresponding levels of development which can be organized through participation in total movement activities. Although these areas are discussed separately, it is hoped that they will nevertheless be seen as interrelated horizontally (among the 16 areas) as well as vertically (within each developmental line). It has been shown that dysfunction in one area affects other areas of psycho-social development. For example, if an individual is unable to organize the ability to be aware of body parts and their relationship (body-image area), he will very probably have a great deal of difficulty shaping his body in relation to the environment (shape area).

It should also be noted that more than one adaptive level may be integrated or organized during a total movement activity. In fact, it is almost impossible to separate related components of the developmental levels of organization if the individual is to be involved in an adequate environment for learning. For example, the therapist could not expect to facilitate the evolution of a patient from investment of positive affect in self and others to investment of aggressive drive in external objects (drive-object area) without the appropriate dyadic relationship. Anna Freud has stated, "If we examine our notions of average normality in detail, we find that we expect a fairly close correspondence between growth on the developmental lines. In clinical terms this means that, to be a harmonious person, a child who has reached a specific stage in the sequence toward emotional maturity, should have attained also corresponding levels in his growth toward bodily independence, in the lines toward companionship, constructive play, etc."[1]

It is also important to clarify the fact that all levels of organization within each of the developmental lines continue throughout life. For example, a person is still aware of the relationship of his body parts after he has organized the ability to nove through space adaptively.[2]

1. Anna Freud, M.D., *Normality and Pathology is Childhood* (New York: International Universities Press, 1966), pp. 84–85.

2. The principles which Erikson utilizes in development apply here:
"(1) Each critical item of psychosocial strength discussed here is systematically related to all others, and they all depend on the proper development in the proper sequence of each item; and (2)Each item exists in some form before its critical time normally arrives." Erik Erikson, *Childhood and Society* (New York: W. W. Norton & Co., 1963), p. 271.

Each developmental line of levels of organization will be divided as follows:

1. A brief summary of the relevance of the developmental levels of organization in Dance-Movement Therapy.
2. A hierarchical outline of the levels of organization.
3. Related maladaptive behavior with suggested methods and techniques for Dance-Movement Therapy.
4. Suggested population for the particular techniques. These will be generally categorized as: adult, child, individual, group, neurotic, and/or psychotic.
5. Related elements: a listing of some related levels of organization from other areas discussed in the chapter.[3]

## TEN BASIC PRINCIPLES

The ten basic principles which will be mentioned here are reminders which will hopefully afford the reader a perspective from which to view the following breakdown of Dance-Movement Therapy areas of concern.

1. Dance-Movement Therapy facilitates more adaptive movement in an individual from the "inside out," not from the "outside in." It is poor reasoning to assume that if an individual does not utilize a particular movement pattern which he needs to live adaptively, the therapist can "teach it" to him.
2. Work from what you see; never superimpose a movement pattern. This is really another way of stating the first principle. Its foundation is based upon a major goal in therapy which is to broaden and enlarge the existing repertoire of an individual for adaptive choices in his life, rather than to try to affix non-idiosyncratic ways of functioning onto his personality.
3. Always consider the particular environment from which the individual comes as well as whether he needs to adapt to new surroundings. For example, to suggest that an American Indian exhibits pathological behavior because he only makes use of directional shape and not shaping as well shows an ignorance which is inexcusable if a therapist is to work with an individual from that culture.

3. Although some of the concepts will not have been previously mentioned, they will be discussed by the end of the chapter. This section was put in only for the therapist or student who intends to use this book as a manual, as its rationale only becomes clear when the reader has read through the chapter at least once. If for example, a client is having difficulty with a particular area, the therapist may make use of related elements to assist the individual in the organization of the component in question.

4. Awareness of the qualities and combinations of attributes which are characteristic of an individual can be a vital and useful tool when working toward the organization of a particular pattern. For example, if a person utilizes directness with slowness and it is desirable to facilitate the exploration and integration of a more aggressive pattern, the following combination might be utilized to evolve the person into a press: directness, slowness, and strength, and gradually as the person becomes comfortable with the addition of this new element of strength, evolve the slowness into acceleration.
5. Awareness of the sequence of a characteristic pattern can also be of importance when working with an individual. If, for example, within the use of tension flow rhythms (which will be discussed in depth later on in the chapter) an individual continually utilizes a particular sequential pattern to work himself up to appropriate expression of anger: (that of oral, oral aggressive, anal sadistic, urethral sadistic, to that of phallic sadistic); the therapist may then make use of this sequence to facilitate the person's experiencing more phallic ballistic patterns.
6. Use of level related components can facilitate organization of a particular element, for example, utilizing related attributes of effort with shape. If an individual has difficulty moving with strength and if a descending pattern is used by him, make use of descending in shaping to aid in the organization of strength.
7. There is always more than one way to aid an individual in the organization of a component. What is best for one may be unsuccessful for another. For example, within the use of metaphor alone there are several alternatives—such as concrete images which may have personal or universal archetypal aspects, sensory images as with sound, sight, or internal kinesthetic improvisations, or abstract images as with expressions of feeling.
8. Remember always that there are levels of organization. To work on kinesthetic discrimination when an individual is unable to respond to any stimulation of this type is fruitless.
9. Generally a therapist can be most assured that an individual has fully organized a particular pattern when he is able to take that pattern throughout his body with his breathing in direct correspondence to the expression, affording an uninterrupted flow of movement. The real tests are of course time, maintenance during stress, and demonstration in appropriate life situations.
10. When feasible it is both expedient and beneficial to make an explicit contract, which determines goals and processes, between therapist

and client/patient(s). It is expedient to the extent that both client/patient(s) and therapist know where they are going; and it is beneficial to the extent that the person(s) shares the responsibility with the therapist, a working alliance being one of the primary goals of the therapeutic relationship.

## FLOW OF BREATH

The most basic of all areas in diagnosis and treatment in Dance-Movement Therapy is the flow of the individual's breathing. It is basic in many ways—first because it is one of the primary indicators of life. From the first scream of breath of the infant to the last gasp of a dying man, the respiratory-circulatory system is the most vital to the physical sustaining and well-being of an individual. Secondly, it is one of the most fundamental behavioral reactions to emotion. Anxiety, anger, and sadness are all reflected in the rate, depth, and facility of breathing. Thirdly, because of the above two factors, it is usually thought of as one of the major agents in assisting the client toward more adaptive functioning.

In *Thus Speaks the Body,* Christensen writes:

"Sucking, biting, chewing, micturition, defecation, orgasm, fear and anger, laughter and grief may all be considered as basic organismic responses, responses having an innate biological source. They are all closely related to respiration. In fact, they may be considered so closely related that unless they become integrated with respiration their expression will neither be complete nore give full release and satiation." (p. 75)

Christensen feels through his experience and study of related research that without the integration and coordination with breathing these so-called organismic responses can neither be learned nor fully organized.

The flow of breath is also considered to be the initiating impulse to the individual's interaction with the environment (both internal and external). Symmetrical shape flow as it is referred to by Lamb and Kestenberg, is characterized by the growing and shrinking of the body during normal breathing. Dr. Kestenberg states: "The rhythm of 'shrinking and growing' provides the motor apparatus for the continuous rhythmic transformation of the narcissistic libido into object libido and vice versa."[4]

Seen in another light, shape flow becomes a basic behavioral reaction to the world outside which corresponds to general feelings of well-being (growing-inhalation) or malaise (shrinking-exhalation).

4. Judith Kestenberg, M.D., *The Role of Movement Patterns in Development* (New York: Dance Notation Bureau, 1966.), p. 88.

## Breath Flow

This area is characterized by the ability to establish total body flow. This occurs when the whole body is allowed to participate actively in the respiratory process. To understand this concept, one must first define normal breathing. Healthy breathing occurs only if the inspiratory and expiratory processes are both complete. Inspiration commences with an outward abdominal movement brought about by the contraction of the diaphragm and the relaxation of the abdominal muscles. This is then followed in a rhythmic fashion by the upward and outward movement of the thorax. In expiration, the reversal of this wave-like rhythmical flow occurs; the chest relaxes, followed by the diaphragm, and then by the abdomen. This flow is primarily felt in the torso and secondarily throughout the whole body. Once this rhythmical flow is achieved at its normal pace, the movement of the individual will become integrated. Organization of the ability to put breathing into the preferred sequence for the desired movement will also be considered here; i.e., breathing must be in the service of movement and expression.

## Related Maladaptive Behavior with Suggested Methods and Techniques for Dance-Movement Therapy: Flow of Breath

A. Maladaptive Behavior: Breathing which is blocked, sporadic, inhibited, or increased to a high anxious rate due to another approaching individual. Fear of another's intrusion or potential demands, projected fantasy that if another would get close enough she would find out how "bad and worthless" he (the patient) really is, and detect a tremendous repressed rage or overwhelming dependency are a few of the possible rationales for this behavior.

Dance-Movement Therapy Techniques:

1. Approach the patient on a diagonal walking in a slow uninterrupted rhythm.
2. With the same flow used in the movement toward the patient, sit quietly beside him as closely as possible without disturbing his proxemic "close space" or kinesphere and imposing a threat on him. (Hall)
3. The posture and mood of the patient must be empathetically reflected in order to be at his level of communication. In this way the person feels that no demands are made on him; he is allowed to be where he feels most comfortable.
4. At the appropriate time which may be after several minutes or several sessions depending on the pathology of the patient and the abilities of the therapist, other forms of communication can begin.

Several methods of communication have proven successful. Flexibility of choice as well as the knowledge of what the most comfortable method is for the therapist himself are two aspects which must be taken into consideration. One method consists of having the therapist verbally or non-verbally offer his hand to the individual. While holding it in a supportive but non-clutching manner, he may begin to rock the hand of the individual gradually including the whole body in the rhythmic flow process. (Chace) Utilizing music which reflects the mood of the relationship with a tempo which simulates that of the breath pulse is often a good idea.[5] Depending on the tactile defensiveness of the individual, the therapist may offer the patient the support of his arms and body in the rocking process.

Once this initial relationship has been established, it becomes a foundation upon which recapitulation of normal developmental organizations and adaptations can take place. Kalish has written, "Following a long period of resistance to any contact, Laura (an autistic child) would go limp and melt into my body as if fused. This seemed to be a physical manifestation of a symbolic relationship. Slowly, over many months, this can change so that the child and therapist can sit and move together as two separate bodies." Janet Adler Boettiger demonstrated a similar progression in her film on Dance Therapy, *Looking for Me.*

The type of approach discussed in this section was evolved by Marian Chace, the founder of Dance Therapy. It was utilized primarily with psychotic individuals, but it has relevance for all ages and all people.

B. Maladaptive Behavior: The maladaptive blocking or immobilization of the chest, diaphragm, abdomen, or pelvis during the breathing process. This then effects the respiration. The blockage usually occurs through the tensing of various muscles in the torso. An example of this is tension in the shoulders or upper back which inhibits the natural reciprocal swing of the arms when walking. The person looks as if he is literally "scared stiff" to "let go." Some psychological interpretations of tension will be given in the chapter on the "Somatatization of Symbols."[6] Another form of blockage, although not as common, is the rendering of the muscles into a flaccid, limp state. The torso is usually lifeless, hollowed, and shortened.

Dance-Movement Therapy Techniques:

1. Movement activities involving the stretching and opening of the chest cavity. For example, hook arms with the individual back-to-back while

5. Music by Erik Satie as well as recorded sounds of the ocean tide have proven successful in this area.

6. Whenever muscles appear to be in a continuous contracted or flaccid state, a possible neuromuscular pathological etiology must be checked out. There are as many physical pathologic causes (e.g., cerebral palsy, Parkinson's disease, cerebral vascular accident, muscular distrophy, etc.) as there are psychological reasons.

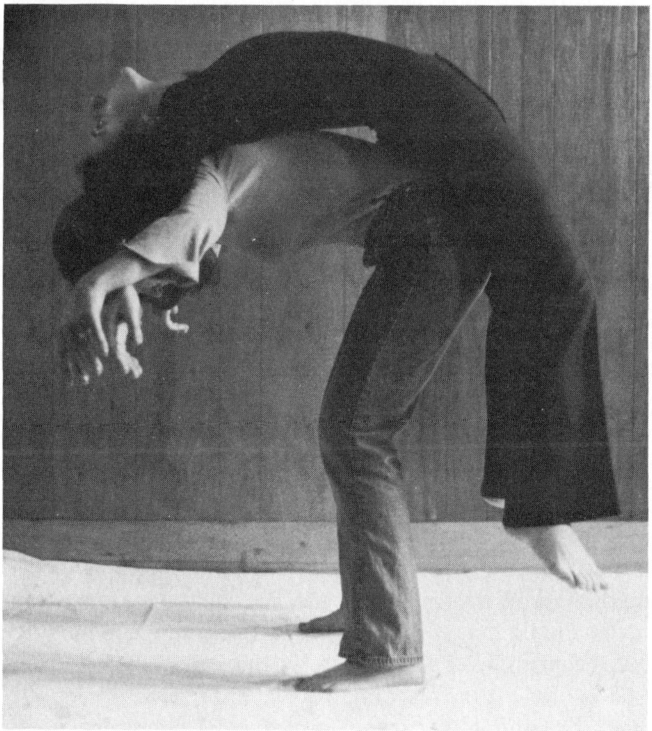

**Figure III.1.** Over the back stretch

standing, and bend forward, lifting him onto your back while pulling his arms away from his chest and letting them hang overhead in a relaxed manner. (Lowen) (See Figure III.1.) Or ask the client to yawn and stretch like a cat, arching his back, extending his legs, loosening and dropping his jaw, and literally "ballooning" himself to occupy the most space possible.[7] (All categories)

2. Movement activities involving the exaggeration of the tense area which is blocking the flow of breathing. This is done in order to produce a safe anxiety state, one in which the individual can become aware of the emotional conflict which has somatatized itself in body tensions, be able to express the emotion he was in conflict about experiencing, and thus bring his resistence into conscious awareness.[8] For example, a young man was

7. Frederick Perls, M.D., Ralph Hefferline, Ph.D., Paul Goodman, Ph.D., *Gestalt Therapy* (New York: Dell & Co., 1957), p. 134.

8. *Ibid.*, p. 287.

not allowing the normal breath pattern of growing and shrinking to occur in his back. The muscles in his upper back were contracted and tense. I suggested to him that he exaggerate the tense area, outline and shape it precisely, and then describe what he was feeling. First, he said it was like a screw digging into his back; he then thought again and said that it was someone's finger jabbing into him. He decided it was his father's finger. His father had always pushed him to do more, be better. The tension was released by a "get off my back" exercise (reciprocal elbow jabs to back). (Neurotics, individuals, adults)

3. Movement activity which allows the patient to cathect the repressed feelings which are producing tensions in his body and inhibiting his breathing process. This will produce emotions such as anger, sadness, fear, and/or joy. This can be done for example, by, evolving the individual into a free flow movement pattern. The therapist may start with swings or any rhythmic pattern in which there is no intention toward any particular dynamics. Then he looks for any possible change of exertion which might be evolving in the patterns of the person. The client may pick up the tempos of the swings or give them more direction than before or incorporate more strength. The therapist may then encourage this pattern either verbally or by duplicating it himself. He will help the individual to heighten the motor expression of the feeling (in this case anger) as well as help the person to level off the response when appropriate. This can be done, for example, by gradually moving toward indirectness in space, lightness in force, and/or deceleration. (See section on effort for more discussion.) (All categories)
4. Movement patterns involving the placement of an individual in various body positions which produce tensions facilitating involuntary movement flow such as those suggested by bioenergists. For example, have the client stand with his feet roughly twelve inches apart while toeing inward. Ask him to bend his knees, lean back, and place his hands at his lower back. (See figure III.2) When the muscles have fatigued sufficiently in this position, the opposing muscle groups will start to coarcate, producing a vibratory undulating rhythm throughout the body.[9] (Neurotics, individuals)
5. Movement activities which involve symbolic imagery as catalysts for movement flow. For example, ask the group to become trees, blades of grass, or flowers moving in the wind. Being swimming fishes or bouncing rag dolls can also be suggested. (All categories)

9. Alexander Lowen, M.D., *The Betrayal of the Body* (New York: The MacMillan Co., 1967).

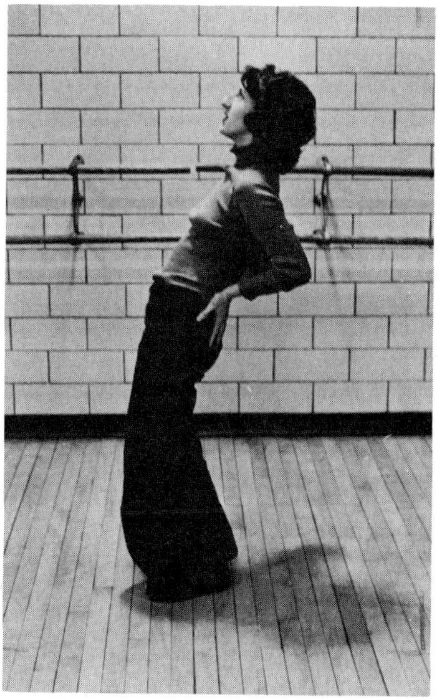

**Figure III.2.**

C. Maladaptive Behavior: Unnatural breathing patterns such as:

1. Incomplete breath flow pattern. (The therapist can easily see whether or not the belly is moving due to the displacement of the diaphragm or if the chest cavity is lengthening, bulging, and/or widening during inhalation.)
2. Lack of adaptive regular even rhythm to the breath flow: for example, if a person is holding his breath during the inhalation or exhalation process or if his flow and/or rate are sporadic.

Dance-Movement Therapy Techniques:

1. Movement activities which stress the breathing process. These are patterns which have a reciprocal in-out, up-down, growing-shrinking sequence. (It is often necessary to remind a person to *breathe fully* and openly no matter what area is being emphasized.)
   a. For example, have the individual lie down on the floor or sit in a chair if the floor is too threatening, and suggest to him that he grow, opening his body when he inhales and shrink, closing himself, when he exhales. (All categories)

b. Another way is to have the clients in a group pair-up holding each others' hands with one seated and one standing. Then instruct them to move in a reciprcal up-down see-saw pattern; i.e., the person standing pulls the seated person (who is inhaling) up to a standing position while be (exhaling) drops to a seated position (Bartenieff). (All categories)

2. Movement patterns which stress regularity of breath flow. For example, the therapist might make use of a record with an even repetitive beat to which a group could alternate a breath flow pattern. (Choose a record which allows for the desired rate of breathing.) (All categories)

3. Moment activities which involve breathing imagery: such as suggesting to the group that they be balloons which blow up and deflate. For exhalation a child could become a melting snowman; for inhalation, a blossoming flower. The therapist should make sure that they inhale and exhale at the appropriate times. (All categories, especially children)

D. Maladaptive Behavior: Unnatural speech. For example, a person's speech is shallow or soft, or he is unable to raise his voice.

Dance-Movement Therapy Techniques: Use of vocalization when moving.

a. For example, suggest to a group that they make nonsensical sounds which might express how they are feeling at the moment. It is easiest to go around a circle at first, giving each person time to make a sound with the contract being that when they feel comfortable, they can respond directly to the sounds that are made. Eventually the whole group joins in. (All categories)

b. An orchestra of sounds can be created while people move to their own "music." (All categories)

c. In individual sessions, clients are sometimes asked, "If your movements could talk, what would they say?" For example, a young woman with whom I was working was getting in touch with some angry feelings as she slashed and punched at a cushion. With the above cue, she started yelling, "Bitch, bitch! Go to hell! You never came, never!" Prior to this incident, she had had no idea that the anger she was releasing each session was due to a deep-seated repression of her mother's inability to meet her needs when she was a child. Because of this awareness, she was able to deal with the cause of her rage and to better understand her relationships with her mother, the therapist, and others. (Adults, neurotics)

## EFFORT-SHAPE LEVELS OF ORGANIZATION

The concepts of effort-shape as devised by Rudolf Laban and Warren Lamb are used to describe and analyze the quality of human movement. When subdivided into the appropriate developmental lines, effort-shape becomes an invaluable tool in Movement Therapy.

Effort can be defined as the way in which kinetic energy is expended in space, force, and time. Within this area, pre-efforts demonstrate the degree of defensiveness of an individual and are utilized in the motor expression of ego defense mechanisms. Efforts serve to subdue and control the flow of tension (discussed in Tension Flow rhythms). They are the adaptive patterns by which the ego controls basic drives such as nurturance, elimination, and sexual gratification. Kestenberg (1979) states that the ego translates the id will (tension flow rhythms) into actions (efforts).

Shape is defined as the form of the movement or how the body changes and moves through space as it adapts to the environment (both human and non-human objects). Directional or dimensional shape is the arc-like or spoke-like bridge between self and objects, while shaping is the three-dimensional system which adds complexity and subtlety to relationships. The flow of shape (shape flow) relates to the differentiation of the self from the object. The qualities of growing and shrinking contribute to the motor apparatus for the discharge of libidinal and aggressive energy from the self to the other which affects the transformation of the narcissistic libido to the object libido (Kestenberg, 1979).

In general, effort-shape is the way in which a person (1) copes with his inner vibrations and (2) makes adaptations in response to the environment (Bartenieff).

Although effort and shape have been divided into separate sub-chapters, they are nevertheless bound together. A brief summary of their relationship will be given at the end of the analysis.[10, 11]

## EFFORT LEVELS OF ORGANIZATION[12]

1. Tension Flow[13]

   This involves the capacity for tension flow which is based on the relationship between the contraction of agonist and antagonist mus-

10. See Appendix for a paralleling of Effort-Shape, Piaget, and Gesell.

11. See Cecily Dell, *A Primer for Movement Description* (New York: Dance Notation Bureau, 1970), for further description of effort-shape concepts as well as use of the notational system.

12. Developmental studies of effort-shape carried out by Dr. Judith Kestenberg. Its application to Dance-Movement Therapy is that of the author.

13. Although tension flow is not by definition an effort quality, it is nevertheless so closely linked with the efforts that it must be considered here. See also Warren Lamb, *Management Behavior* (New York: International Universities Press, 1969); and Warren Lamb and Elizabeth Watson, *Body Code* (London: Routledge and Kegan Paul, 1979).

cles. This flow is either bound (greater participation of antagonists) or free (greater participation of agonists). Id drive discharge rhythms of tension flow can be present at birth; however, due to lack of psycho-physiologic maturation and/or environmental stimuli, organization of them may not yet be achieved. Thus, the flow is unstabilized, undifferentiated and not yet organized to a particular zone.

2. Primal Regulation of Tension Flow

   The primal regulation of tension flow involves the ability to distinguish between continuity and discontinuity of motility. It requires the ability to initiate, continue, and cessate basic reflexive movement patterns such as sucking and grasping and reflects the capacity for id discharge of drives.

3. Spatial Pre-effort

   This involves the ability to cope with the external forces of space using changes in tension. It requires the ability to change one's mental state to respond to the environment, either by *channeling* movement which is accomplished by the use of even flow tension, and/or by moving with *flexibility* which is achieved by adjusting the flow of tension.

4. Gravitational or Weight Pre-effort

   This involves the ability to cope with the external forces of gravity using changes in tension. It requires the ability to change one's mental state to respond to the environment, either by moving with *vehemence* which is accomplished by the use of a high intensity of tension, and/or by moving with *gentleness* which is accomplished by the use of a low intensity of tension.

5. Time Pre-effort

   This involves the ability to cope with the external forces of time using changes in tension. It requires the ability to change one's mental state to respond to the environment, either by moving with *suddenness* which is accomplished by the use of a steep ascent of tension, and/or by moving with *hesitation* which is accomplished by the use of a gradual descent of tension.

6. Spatial Effort

   This involves the habitual and automatic adaptive pattern which is utilized to cope with the spatial factors of the environment. It requires the ability to utilize *indirect* movement in which spatial attention consists of overlapping shifts in the body among a number of foci, and *direct* movement in which spatial attention in the body is a pinpointed single focus (Dell). These efforts relate to the capacity to investigate and define (Lamb, Ramsden). With the organization of this level comes the ability to attend to a situation. This pattern, like all of the following efforts, extends to fine as well as gross movements.

7. Gravitational or Weight Effort

   This involves the habitual and automatic adaptive pattern which is utilized to cope with weight factors in the environment. This level of organization requires the ability to increase pressure of body weight to a forceful degree entailing the use of *strength* and the ability to withhold and rarefy the feeling of weight entailing the use of *lightness* (Dell). These qualities correspond with the capacity to persist with determination, to have commitment and conviction (Lamb, Ramsden). With the organization of this level comes the ability to discipline with firmness or sensitivity in intention.[14]

8. Time Effort

   This level of organization involves the habitual and automatic adaptive pattern which is utilized to cope with the temporal factors in the environment. It requires the ability to move with urgency or quickening in time in *acceleration* and the ability to prolong or stretch out movement in *deceleration.* Being able to decide with a sense of timing as well as the capacity to carryout a task is associated with these dynamics (Lamb, Ramsden). With the organization of this pattern comes the ability to make a decision on a commitment.[15]

9. Incomplete Efforts and Inner Attitudes[16]

   This involves the ability to combine two of the four elements of space, weight, time, and flow to produce an incomplete effort. This form of organization reveals "inner states of mind" or inner attitudes. The possible combinations are listed here.

   a. Weight and flow—"dreamlike, creative or doubting, restrictive"
      1. strong and bound—"cramped with tension"
      2. strong and free—"firm, 'easy' flow"
      3. light and bound—"delicate, with great care"
      4. light and free—"flying, buoyant"

14. *Ibid.*

15. *Ibid.*

16. Abstracted from Marian North, *Personality Assessment Through Movement* (London: MacDonald & Evans, Ltd., 1972), pp. 246–255.

b. Space and flow—"remote"
   1. direct and bound—"controlled"
   2. direct and free—"fluent, channeled"
   3. indirect and bound—"knotting"
   4. indirect and free—"undulating"

c. Time and flow—"adaptability, mobility"
   1. sudden and bound—"jerky"
   2. sudden and free—"bouncy, urgent"
   3. sustained and bound—"cautious"
   4. sustained and free—"unharried, lazy"

d. Space and time—"awake"
   1. direct and sudden—"sharp, tapping"
   2. direct and sustained—"smooth"
   3. indirect and sudden—"fluttering"
   4. indirect and sustained—"slow twisting"

e. Weight and time—"earthiness"
   1. strong and sudden—"forceful, energetic"
   2. strong and sustained—"powerful, persevering"
   3. light and sudden—"lively, delicate"
   4. light and sustained—"peaceful, soothing"

f. Weight and space—"stability"
   1. strong and direct—"firm, commanding"
   2. strong and indirect—"sinuous, striving"
   3. light and direct—"gently pointed"
   4. light and indirect—"sensitive"

10. Externalized Drives

This form of organization involves the ability to automatically combine three elements involving the attributes of space, weight, time, and/or flow in order to fully adapt to ego based reality cope with the total environment. This requires the appropriate body-movement organization for:

a. Action—flowless
   1. light, slow, indirect—float
   2. light, quick, direct—dab
   3. light, slow, direct—glide

4. light, quick, indirect—flick
5. strong, quick, direct—punch
6. strong, quick, indirect—slash
7. strong, slow, direct—press
8. strong, slow, indirect—wring

b. Passion—spaceless[17]
1. strong, quick, bound—"possessive, aggressive"
2. strong, quick, free—"uncontrolled, wild"
3. strong, slow, bound—"restrictive"
4. strong, quick, free—"outgoing, powerful ease"
5. light, quick, bound—"little irritations"
6. light, quick, free—"flippant"
7. light, slow, bound—"hesitant, shy"
8. light, slow, free—"indulging, formless"

c. Vision—weightless
1. direct, quick, bound—"penetrating"
2. direct, quick, free—"lively reactions"
3. direct, slow, bound—"slow penetration of restricted idea"
4. direct, slow, free—"continued pursuance of clear aim"
5. indirect, quick, bound—"controlled sudden avoidance"
6. indirect, quick, free—"sudden imaginative ideas"
7. indirect, slow, bound—"cautious"
8. indirect, slow, free—"imaginative indulging"

d. Spell—timeless
1. direct, strong, bound—"concentration"
2. direct, strong, free—"resolute drive for power"
3. direct, light, bound—"tentative, meticulous"
4. direct, light, free—"clear direction"
5. indirect, strong, bound—"restricted"
6. indirect, strong, free—"generous, influencing"
7. indirect, light, bound—"uncertain restraint"
8. indirect, light, free—"yielding to influence"

17. *Ibid.*, pp. 263–266.

## Related Maladaptive Behavior with Suggested Methods and Techniques for Dance-Movement Therapy

1. Tension Flow

   Maladaptive Behavior:[18] Predominance of neutral flow throughout the body such that there is little or no reversal from free to bound flow or vice versa.

   Dance-Movement Therapy Techniques:

   1. Movement activities which involve an evolutionary development of flow fluctuations (free-bound alternation). Depending on the patient, movement can flow from proximal to distal, cephalo to caudal, from the center of gravity-out or the reverse. Whichever is the most basic and/or least threatening should be centered on first.

      For example, some severely regressed schizophrenic individuals seem only to allow movement to occur on a distal (i.e., only lower arm and lower leg) level. The therapist may take this cue and suggest to the patient to move these parts in a rhythmic flow pattern. He may then gradually suggest to him to involve the more proximal parts of the body.

      On other occasions the individual must first get a sense of the center of gravity via such basic patterns as sitting, standing, being on "all-fours," and tilting the body and regaining balance. Once this awareness has developed he may feel more comfortable rocking in a flow pattern alternating his center stance (Bartenieff). (All categories, particularly the organically dysfunctioned)

   2. Movement activities involving the development of involuntary coarcation of muscles (Lowen). This quick abrupt change from free to bound flow can then be exaggerated to produce flow throughout the body.

      For example, suggest to the person that he stand in a parallel position, his legs about eight inches apart, and his knees bent to produce roughly a 130° angle. Due to muscle fatigue, the upper leg muscles' [agonists (quadraceps) and antagonists

18. It is important to remember when viewing so-called maladaptive behavior that absence of movement elements are not necessarily pathological. Their absence may facilitate an individual's functioning at a particular job or in a cultural environment. Behavior becomes maladaptive only when the person cannot satisfy his own needs and meet the demands of the environment. Therefore, the behavior must always be considered in relation to the cultural-socio-economic profile of the individual.

(hamstrings)] holding contractions will become more pronounced producing a shaking motion. Suggest to the person that he take this rhythm into his whole body. (Neurotics, adults, individuals, groups)

3. Movement activities involving the use of imagery. For example, instruct the group to become giggling motors. (Children)

Related elements which will be discussed in later chapters are the utilization of enactive, iconic, or abstract cognition,[19] one-to-one or parallel group,[20] use of egocentric or object-dependent relationship with therapist,[21] and use of symmetrical shape flow.[22]

2. Primal Regulation of Tension Flow

A. Maladaptive Behavior: Difficulty in distinguishing between preserving and establishing movement flow.

Dance-Movement Therapy Techniques:

Suggest to the person that he move and cease movement. Use of graded sensory reinforcements may be required.

For example, have the person sit or stand in front of a mirror (visual cue); touch his arm and ask him to move it (tactile cue and verbal cue). You may wish also to weight the arm or body part. The same procedure may be used when asking the person to stop moving. The extra stimuli may be reduced when the individual is ready. (All categories including retarded individuals, but usually not applicable to neurotics)

B. Maladaptive Behavior: Difficulty in adaptively initiating, continuing, and cessating basic movement patterns.

Dance-Movement Therapy Techniques:

Movement activities which facilitate the starting and stopping of patterns.

For example, use such games as "freeze": the group is allowed to move until the therapist instructs them to freeze at which time they hold their positions. (Children, individuals, groups, neurotics, psychotics, organically dysfunctioned)

Related elements which will be discussed later are one-to-one, parallel group, object ambivalent or semi-autonomous relationship with therapist, and the use of symmetrical shape flow.

19. Will be discussed in detail in the Cognitive Representation Levels of Organization.
20. Will be discussed in detail in the Primary Group Levels of Organization.
21. Will be discussed in detail in the Dyadic Levels of Organization.
22. Will be discussed in detail in the Shape Levels of Organization.

3. Spacial Pre-effort

A. Maladaptive Behavior: Difficulty in adaptively coping with the external forces of space through appropriate channeling. This characterizes a person, for example, who has difficulty restricting himself to one thing at a time; he cannot get the appropriate mental feeling about moving in an even manner in space. This behavior may also characterize a person who uses flexibility through deflection, avoidance, or intellectualization as a predominant defense mechanism.

Dance-Movement Therapy Techniques.

1. Movement activities involving a conscious effort to maintain even flow in moving through space. The therapist can assist this process by reminding the person to channel his body and by keeping him centered on his bodily felt experience and associated emotions rather than intellectual discussions and analyses which separate him from the soma. (All categories)
2. Movement activity in which the person reinforces channeling by a verbal stream of consciousness. The therapist might suggest that he focus on a continuum of body awareness; i.e., "Now I am aware of . . ." (All categories)

B. Maladaptive Behavior: Difficulty in coping with the external forces of space through appropriate flexibility. This might characterize an individual who is over-cautious or who is restraining when he should be more able to adjust himself, or it may describe someone who uses channeling through isolation or emotional insulation as his predominant defense mechanism.

Dance-Movement Therapy Techniques:

1. Movement activities involving a conscious adjustment of flow of tension in moving through space.

   For example, the therapist keeps suggesting to the person that he think about being more flexible when moving in space, indulge himself, allow himself to take in as much space as possible. His own verbal cues may also help. (All categories with change of vocabulary)

2. Movement activities which foster relatedness with other group members. Suggest such activities as, "find different ways of greeting people using different body parts." (All categories)

   Related elements are: one-to-one, parallel group, object ambivalent or semi-autonomous relationship with therapist, use of horizontal directional shape.

4. Gravitational or Weight Pre-effort

   Maladaptive Behavior: Difficulty in coping with the external forces of weight through the appropriate use of vehemence and/or gentleness. This might characterize a person who maladaptively overuses gentleness to the extent that he becomes too vague, serving the defense mechanism of reaction formation, or who overuses vehemence such that he feels cramped and static all the time as in the defense mechanism of defensive stubbornness or identification with the aggressor.

   Dance-Movement Therapy Techniques:

   Movement activities involving a conscious effort to maintain high-intensity flow and/or low-intensity flow.

   1. Movement dramas which involve the polar roles of aggressor and victim as well as the exploration of the continuum between these two opposite roles. (All categories)
   2. Movement improvisations which entail the exaggeration of vehement stubbornness, hopefully resulting in eventual homeostatic relaxation. (All categories)

   Related elements are: one-to-one, parallel groups, object ambivalent or semi-autonomous relationship with therapist, use of vertical directional shape.

5. Time Pre-effort

   Maladaptive Behavior: Difficulty in adaptively coping with the external forces of time through the appropriate use of suddenness and/or hesitation. This state might be exemplified by a man who uses suddenness in service to the ego defense mechanism of escape or hesitation in counter phobic behavior. (All categories)

   Dance-Movement Therapy Techniques:

   1. Movement activities involving a conscious effort to maintain suddenness and/or hesitation. The therapist gives verbal cues. (All categories)
   2. Patterns involving alternation of these two qualities.

   For example, involve the person in consciously feeling a slow deliberateness of movement juxtaposed with one in which he readies his state for quick sudden patterns. The therapist may wish to have the person sense the difference without moving, followed by taking this movement into space. Re-enactments of that which is anxiety-provoking along with the exploration of the polar time pre-effort may facilitate adaptivity. (All categories)

Related elements are: one-to-one, parallel group, object-ambivalent or semi-autonomous relationship with therapist, use of sagittal directional shape.

6. Spacial Effort

A. Maladaptive Behavior: Difficulty in moving with directness when adaptively appropriate. This could manifest itself in an individual with an exaggerated predominant use of indirectness. The person would lack focus, be all over the place without any real purpose, and have a great deal of difficulty sticking to any task.

Dance-Movement Therapy Techniques:

Gross and fine movement patterns involving the use of directness. The therapist can utilize imagery or create an actual environment which requires the person to make use of the particular dynamic, in this case directness.

For example, the therapist could suggest to a group that there is a very narrow bridge over some water in front of them and that they should walk across being careful not to fall off. (All categories)

Related element: Use of narrowing shaping.

B. Maladaptive Behavior: Difficulty in moving with indirectness when adaptively appropriate. A person might be too narrow and meticulous, unable to take in the full range of space.

Dance-Movement Therapy Techniques:

Gross and fine movement patterns involving the use of indirectness.

For example, suggest to the individual that there is a field of flowers in front of him and that he wants to take in all of them, and that not being in any hurry he can indulge this desire. (All categories)

The therapist might use an obstacle course of objects which keeps a person from going straight to the other side of the room, but rather permits him to move through space in a meandering pattern. (All categories)

Related elements: Use of widening shaping plus object ambivalent or semi-autonomous relationship, and parallel or task group.

7. Gravitational of Weight Effort

A. Maladaptive Behavior: Difficulty in moving with strength when adaptively appropriate. A person with this problem might be over-sensitive, lacking the feeling of having his feet on the ground, and demonstrating very little drive.

Dance-Movement Therapy Techniques;

The engagement of the person in moving with strength in gross and fine movements.

The therapist might suggest to the client that he walk at his own pace and, utilizing the time and space element with which he feels most comfortable, take a firmer step, perhaps using the imagery of stamping out.

Related element: sinking in shaping.

B. Maladaptive Behavior: Difficulty in moving with lightness when adaptively appropriate. This could characterize a person who uses an excessive amount of strength with little or no rebound into lightness. He may be stubborn to the point of being cramped and immobile; he may be aggressively dogmatic with others.

Dance-Movement Therapy Techniques:

Movement activities involving the use of lightness in gross and fine patterns.

The person might be taken through a fantasy of having a huge weight lifted off his shoulders while he is moving at his own pace about the room.

(Stress the incorporation of as many qualities within his existing repertoire as possible. For example, if the individual always makes use of directness with strength, combine the directness with the experiences of lightness as well.) (All categories)

Related elements: Use of rising shaping as well as parallel or task groups, semi-autonomous, object-ambivalent relationship.

8. Time Effort Stage

A. Maladaptive Behavior: Difficulty in accelerating when adaptively appropriate. This person might be very slow in making decisions wanting to cling to what has existed in the past.

Dance-Movement Therapy Techniques:

Movement activity involving the use of acceleration in gross and fine movements.

For example, throw a ball to the individual and suggest to him that it is "a hot potato" and for him to quickly throw it back. Or suggest to a group that they might dart and stop here and there throughout the room as if they were birds escaping from a net. (All categories)

The therapist might make use of the attributes of space, force, and/or flow to provide a comfortable base for acceleration. The increase in tempo can be gradual, such as with the theme from *Zorba the Greek,* or much quicker such as with a change of a song.

Related element: Use of retreating in shaping.

B. Maladaptive Behavior: Difficulty in decelerating when adaptively appropriate. For example, someone might be unable to slow down such that he is over-hasty about decisions and demonstrates reckless behavior.

Dance-Movement Therapy Techniques:

Movement activity involving the use of deceleration in gross and fine movement.

The therapist might have the group move in an atmosphere filled with glue or underwater, or suggest to a person that he slowly go up to the sleeping monster and then jump on him (children). (All categories)

Related elements: Use of advancing in shaping plus parallel or task groups, object-ambivalent or semi-autonomous relationship with therapist.

9. Incomplete Efforts and Inner Attitudes

A. Maladaptive Behavior: Difficulty in utilizing a two-effort quality when adaptively appropriate.

Dance-Movement Therapy Techniques:

1. Movement activity which makes use of existing repertoire of inner attitudes to evolve the individual toward organization of the two-effort pattern desired.

For example, supposing the therapist senses that a person lacks a feeling of stability (weight and space), and that he seems to always be in a far-off remote state (space and flow). The therapist could then utilize his pre-existing organization of space and, if his disposition in flow is free, gradually evolve him into a straightforward (directness) sensitivity (lightness) which produces a gentle steadfastness. Once this is a comfortable state, the therapist may wish to evolve him into a more solid pattern through evolution into strength with directness. (All categories)

2. Movement activities which involve forms of dancing and which are related to the incomplete efforts. For example, the therapist might suggest African music such as the *Misa Luba* or Olatungi to get in touch with weight-time factors' whereas space-flow, its opposite, fits better with classical ballet. Weight-space is more characteristic of American Indian dances.[23] (All categories when ready)

3. Movement-drama activities which call for the dancing out of an attitude, image, or many attitudes through the use of appropriate character or symbols.

   For example, suggest, concepts such as exuberance (strength-free flow), dogmatic (strength-suddenness), or carefree (indirect-free), or images such as a fluttering butterfly (quick-indirect) or a prowling panther (strength-flexibility).

B. Maladaptive Behavior: Maladaptive exaggeration of a two-effort inner attitude.[24]

   Such as:

   a. Weight and flow
      1. strong and bound—"obsessional, fixated, nightmarish"
      2. strong and free—"overbearing, reckless"
      3. light and bound—"oversensitive, overcautious"
      4. light and free—"unfocused drifting"

   b. Space and flow
      1. direct and bound—"withdrawing, very narrow view of problem"
      2. direct and free—"overemotional, without caution"
      3. indirect and bound—"gets cramped trying to cope with too many aspects at once"
      4. indirect and free—"can't stick to the point, attention swamped by feelings"

   c. Time and flow
      1. quick and bound—"hasty jump to conclusion, inhibited"
      2. quick and free—"rushing at decision"

23. North, *Ibid.*
24. *Ibid.*

3. slow and bound—"cramped"
4. slow and free—"excessively sentimental"

d. Space and time
   1. direct and quick—"narrow-minded"
   2. direct and slow—"clinging to limited view"
   3. indirect and quick—"agitated, anxious"
   4. indirect and slow—"vague, lazy"

e. Weight and time
   1. strong and quick—"domineering, impatient"
   2. strong and slow—"boring insistence"
   3. light and quick—"fleeting intention"
   4. light and slow—"can't come to grips with self"

f. Weight and space
   1. strong and direct—"stubborn, unimaginative"
   2. strong and indirect—"grinding, always changing focus"
   3. light and direct—"superficial, attention to the little detail"
   4. light and indirect—"butterfly mind, meandering"

Dance-Movement Therapy Techniques:

1. Movement patterns involving the gradual evolvement away from the exaggerated degree by movement toward the use of the reciprocal quality.

   For example, if a person over-uses bound coupled with direct, it will manifest itself as a controlled over-cautiousness which might result in, or be a part of a withdrawal reaction. Maintaining the directness, the boundness is gradually relaxed through the involvement in direct-free patterns. Upbeats and rebounds into free before and after a direct-bound pattern will also assist in releasing him from the continuous use of this pattern. (All categories)

2. Movement improvisations using dialogues between personified aspects of the person's psychology which reflect polar qualities. (All categories, particularly neurotic)

   Related elements: Use of corresponding shape affinities, parallel or task group, semi-autonomous or chumship relationship.

10. Externalized Drives

Maladaptive Behavior: Difficulty in utilizing a three-effort combination when adaptively appropriate. Resistances which result in an inability to fully employ ego motor apparatuses for the mediation of drive discharge. For example, a young woman who has trouble expressing her anger is unable to combine directness, strength, and acceleration to produce a punch. The closest she would come to it would be a bound, indirect, accelerated gesture.

Dance-Movement Therapy Techniques:

1. Movement activities which evolve the group or individual from one externalized drive into another.

   For example, if the woman referred to above were to work with a dance therapist, he might suggest to her either verbally by showing her, and/or by taking her through the pattern, to evolve the indirectness to directness producing a quick, direct, bound pattern. The boundness might then be relaxed more into a free-bound alternation or with time the therapist might carefully introduce strength to produce the action of punching. (All categories)

   Quite often when a person is frightened of the heightened agressive expression of a punch, a press (strong, direct, and sustained) might be introduced as less threatening. The therapist might suggest that the person press against his palms as he presses against the client's. A fuller working through of this somatically manifested conflict occurs when the underlying resistances are revealed and the developmental etiology for the maladaptive pattern is uncovered.

2. Movement activities which make use of imagery such as flicking off water (light, indirect, quick), slashing wood in two with a sword (strong, indirect, quick,) or floating along with a cloud having all the time in the world (light, sustained, indirect). (All categories)

3. Movement activities involving gradually or quickly evolving the whole body into an externalized drive.

   For example, suggest to a group that they flick off imaginary water with their hands, then whole arms, arms and shoulders, upper torso, etc. (All categories)

   Sometimes it is more effective to quickly involve a client into a full effort sequence. An example of this phenomenon is a

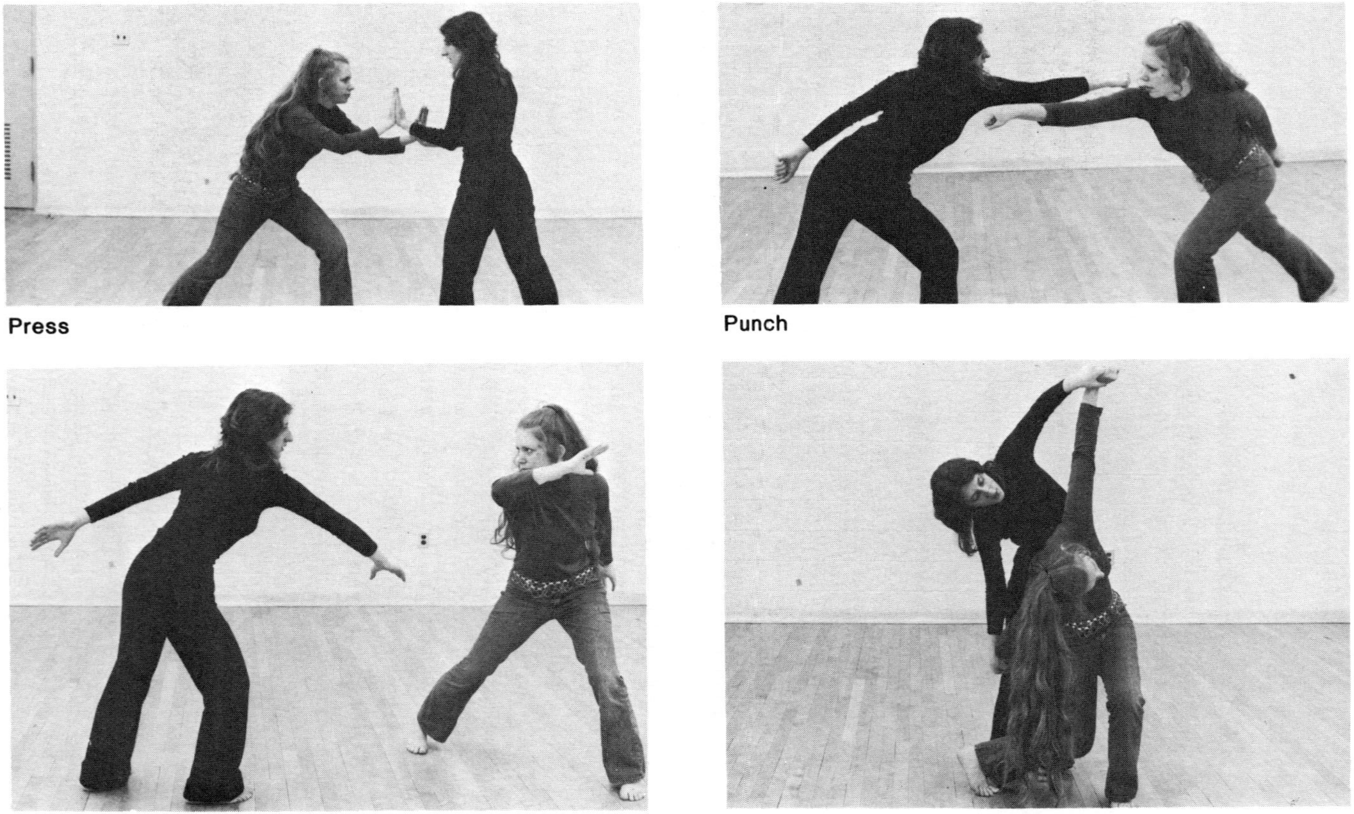

Press

Punch

Slash

Wring

**Figure III.3.** Fighting efforts

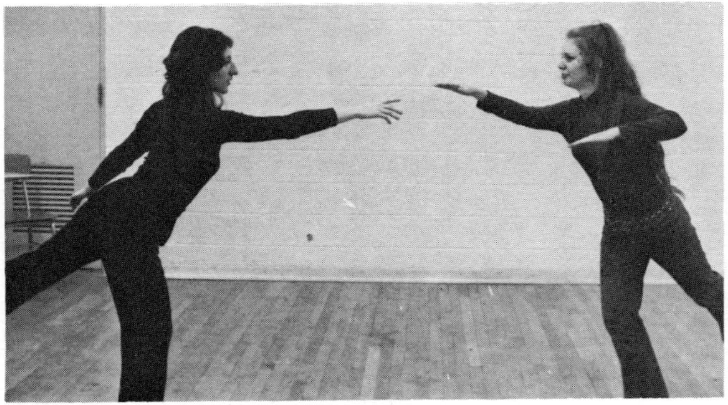

Glide

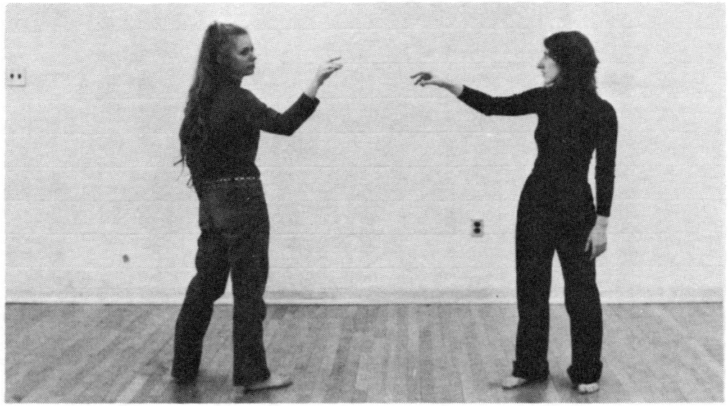

Flick

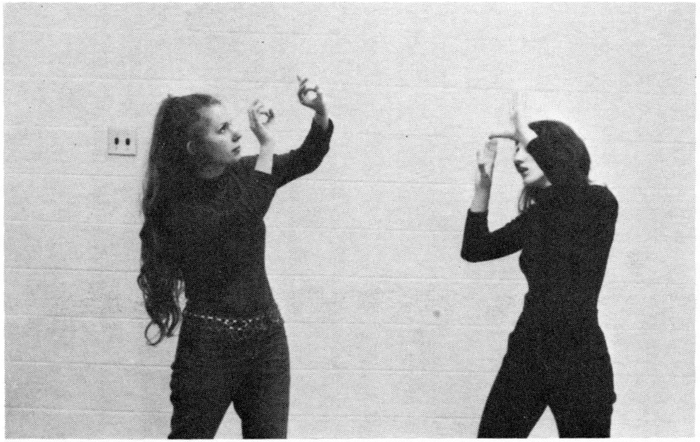

Dab

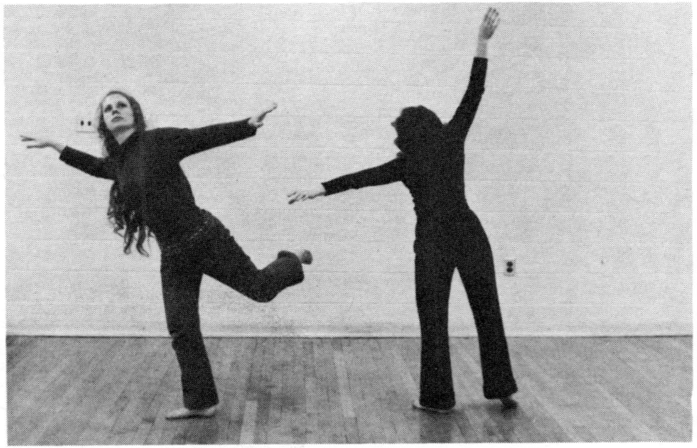

Float

Figure III.4. Indulging efforts

situation in which a catatonic schizophrenic was sliding into a split. The therapist instructed him to "stamp your feet!" (use of a punch: strong, quick, direct, full effort). He immediately got out of his static state and began vigorously stamping. (Following this session, he began taking for the first time since his stay at the day hospital) (Bartenieff). (Catatonic psychotic individuals)

Related elements: Use of all related shape combinations; task, egocentric, and/or cooperative groups; semi-autonomous, chumship or autonomous relationship with the therapist.

## SHAPE LEVELS OF ORGANIZATION[25]

1. Symmetrical Shape Flow

This involves the capacity for spontaneous symmetrical shape flow which is based on the alternation of growing and shrinking of the body in bipolar form. Shape flow is part of the congenital motor equipment which evenually is used by the individual in his attempts to relate to the atmosphere. In affinities, shape flow is characterized by a transition from free flow extensor dominance to bound flow flexor dominance. In general, when an individual grows in shape, body boundaries subside and the feeling is one of expansiveness, generosity, pride, pleasure, and satiation—of wanting to take in the environment. Conversely when an individual shrinks and closes himself from the environment the feeling is associated with affectual sensations such as hunger, pain, despair, as well as retreat from the surroundings. The person may feel himself to be small, empty, or insignificant as compared to his surround. These global affectual responses to objects reach ascendancy during the symbiotic phase of object relationship development (Mahler, 1968).

Shape flow must occur in three dimensions in order for it to be considered fully organized.

Width-widening (expanding, taking in), narrowing (constricting)

Height—lengthening (extending, elongating), shortening (becoming smaller)

Depth—bulging (feeling full), hollowing (feeling empty)

2. Asymmetrical Shape Flow

This involves the capacity for asymmetrical changes in shape which are based on the alternation of growing and shrinking of the body

25. Concepts formulated by Kestenberg.

in unipolar or asymmetrical form. With this apparatus, the individual is able to react to discrete stimuli and to discriminate between what is satisfying and what is repulsive. He is also capable of relating to the space inside his body as well as that which is outside in his immediate near space. Relatedness to external objects is more specified and delineated via "channels" for tension flow rhythms. This adaptive pattern serves secondary narcissism and the rapprochement subphase of Mahler's separation-individuation process. Assymmetrical shape flow reflects the shift from the primary symbiotic dependent state with the maternal object to a greater reliance upon the functioning of the libidinally cathected ego (Mahler, 1968).

In order for this ability to be considered fully organized, the individual must have in his repertoire all the following shape components:

Widening into and out of

Narrowing into and out of

Lengthening up and down

Shortening up and down

Bulging forward and backward

Hollowing forward and backward

3. Horizontal Directional Shape

This involves the capacity of automatic spoke-like or arc-like shaping of the body in space in the horizontal direction. At this level the body or parts of the body is (are) capable of expanding horizontally *sideways* and *across the body* in response to the environment and its objects. This ability is related to the pre-effort stage of channeling and being flexible and is in dominance during the oral phase.

4. Vertical Directional Shape

This involves the capacity for automatic spoke-like or arc-like shaping of the body in space through the vertical dimension. At this level, the body or body parts is (are) capable of extending vertically *upwards* and *downwards* in response to the environment and its objects. This ability is related to the pre-effort stage of gentleness and vehemance and is in dominance during the anal phase.

5. Sagittal Directional Shape

This involves the capacity for automatic spoke-like or arc-like shaping of the body in space in the sagittal dimension. At this level, the body or body parts is (are) capable of protruding *forwards* and *backwards* in response to the environment and its objects. This ability is related to the pre-effort stage of hesitation and suddenness and is in dominance during the urethral phase.

6. Horizontal Shaping

   This involves the capacity for automatic shaping of the body in space utilizing the horizontal plane. This is accomplished by projecting the body or body parts in a *spreading* and *enclosing* shaping of space. These qualities are associated with the ability to explore the shape of possibilities within a given situation and when matched with the effort spatial affinities demonstrate an ability to establish and maintain reciprocal communication and to attend to the environment (Lamb, Ramsden).

7. Vertical Shaping

   This involves the capacity for automatic shaping of the body in space utilizing the vertical plane. This is accomplished by projecting the body or body parts in an *ascending* and *descending* shaping of space. This is the plane of confrontation and intention. The effort affinities are lightness and strength and when appropriately combined with corresponding qualities in shaping result in the ability to present self and others and to influence and persuade while maintaining a sense of confidence and intention.

8. Sagittal Shaping

   This involves the capacity for automatic shaping of the body in space utilizing the sagittal plane. This is accomplished by projecting the body or body parts in an *advancing* and *retreating* shaping of space. This is the plane of anticipation and farsightedness and involves the ability to be committed. When combined with the effort affinities of slowness and quickness, the capacity to carry out plans or "operate" is manifested (Lamb, Ramsden).

9. Combination of Two Qualities in Shaping

   This requires the ability to combine shaping automatically in two planes to cope with either the communicational-presentational, communicational-operational, or operational-presentational situations in the environment.

10. Combination of Three Qualities in Shaping

    This involves the ability of the individual to automatically combine three elements in shaping and involves aspects necessary for comminication, presentation, and operation in order to cope with the spatial environment. It must be remembered that transition from one plane to another requires a shaping movement involving three spatial tendencies. At this level the individual must be able not only to move peripherially, but also transversally (movement which passes between the body center and periphery) as well as centrally (movement which passes through the center of the body).

At this point shape flow is seen as being in total service of shaping[26] in creating the inner as well as outer shape.

## Related Maladaptive Behavior with Suggested Methods and Techniques for Dance-Movement Therapy

1. Symmetrical Shape Flow

A. Maladaptive Behavior: Difficulty in adaptive usage of symmetrical shape flow in any of the three dimensions. What is quite characteristic of many individuals who wish to withdraw from reality is a predominantly fixed position comprised of solely narrowing, shortening, and/or hollowing. Minimal breathing occurs so as not to disturb this body attitude.

Dance-Movement Therapy Techniques:

1. Appropriate movement activities of the flow of breath area. See pp. 12–18; for example: those techniques utilized to promote normal breath flow.
2. Movement activities which stress work on the separate elements of shape flow with the idea of combining them once the person has organized them. For example, suggest to the person that he lie down on the floor. If he uses primarily space efforts or horizontal shape, the therapist may wish to first work on the widening and narrowing of the body during the breath flow, i.e., having the client widen when inhaling and narrow when exhaling. If the client needs more help in understanding and organizing this process, the therapist may wish to use a mirror, show the person his own body, touch the area to be worked on by pressing during exhalation, ask the person to "breathe into my hands" or "breathe into the direction of my hands" during inhalation, or move various body parts. Anxiety may emerge as

26. Shaping in movement involves the changing of three dimensional relationships of the body to space and objects. Kinesthetically, shaping requires flexion or extension, abduction or adduction, and internal or external rotation. Shape flow must be able to be in the control of the individual so as to be put into the preferred sequence for the desired movement; e.g., when an individual spreads his body, he might also wish to widen in shape flow.

somatic pockets of conflict are awakened. "Working through" through identification and re-experiencing of developmentally based maladaptive patterns and trauma is required for integration of this adaptive behavior. (All categories)

3. Dance activities which make use of atmospheric imagery. For example, say, "It's a beautiful day. You are very much alive and filled with joy. Take in your surroundings." (All categories)

B. Maladaptive Behavior: Fixation or regression to the autistic phase of development resulting in a lifeless deanimated body in relation to primary objects.

Dance-Movement Therapy Techniques:

Movement activities which develop symbiotic object relationship with the therapist and the establishment or restoration of a sense of entity and body-image identity (Mahler, 1968). A researched technique is Siegel's (1978) "breathing together" in which therapist and child sit facing each other with the therapist's hand placed over the child's hand on the patient's chest and the child's other hand over the therapist's remaining hand on the therapist's chest. The therapist and child breathe in synchrony and a full bipolar growing and shrinking in symbiotic dual unity is encouraged.[27]

Related elements: Flow of breath; enactive level of cognition; egocentric relationship with therapist, positive affect investment in body.

2. Asymmetrical Shape Flow

A. Maladaptive Behavior: Difficulty in the adaptive usage of asymmetrical shape flow in any of the dimensions. For example, a psychotic child may not have fully organized the ability to grow asymmetrically toward a positive stimulus due to lack of fully integrating the symbiotic phase of development. Any experience of beginning separateness might overwhelm the brittle ego bringing about an annihilation panic. To move toward or away from an object presupposes initial differentiation.

Dance-Movement Therapy Techniques:

1. Movement activities which promote discrimination between and appropriate shape flow responses to inner enteroceptive sensa-

27. The stages of development referred to in this section are those of object relations theorist, Margaret Mahler (1968). They are as follows: normal autism (0–1 month), an undifferentiated matrix of mother/child; symbiosis (2–5 months), a mother/child omnipotent system of dual unity which culminates in beginning self object differentiation; separation-individuation (6–30 months), with subphases of practicing (moving out and returning to mother) and rapprochement (need for mother to share in every experience); and finally, object constancy, mother is internalized.

tions and outer stimuli. The therapist acts as an ego buffer and helps the child distinguish between inner and outer (Mahler, 1968). (Autistic, childhood psychosis, adult psychosis)

2. Movement activities which involve discrimination between attractive and repulsive stimuli. For example, the individual is asked to imagine two stimuli, one positive to be approached and one negative to be withdrawn from. (All categories) With children, the therapist might have the child select two puppets to personify the characteristics.

B. Maladaptive Behavior: A continuous maladaptive asymmetrical body stance.

Dance-Movement Therapy Techniques:

Movement activities which promote normal symmetrical flow of breath through the use of various cues. For example:

a. Use of touch: The therapist alternates pressing and releasing the contracted shrunken side in the rhythm of the person's flow of breath.

b. Use of pre-efforts and efforts: For example, use of lightness to release a shortening down to a lengthening upward or strength to release a shortening up to a lengthening downward.

c. Use of efforts with flow: For example, suggest that the person make use of bound strength in the asymmetrically shrunken area to be released into free strength after a period of time.

d. Use of sound: For example, suggest to the person that he increase the bound flow in the area followed by a sound producing release. (All categories)

Related elements: Flow of breath, enactive and iconic levels of cognition, primal regulation of tension flow; object-ambivalent relationship with therapist; one-to-one, or parallel group.

3. Horizontal Directional Shape[28]

Maladaptive Behavior: Difficulty in adaptively moving in an arc-like or spoke-like manner in the horizontal, such as an individual who has not perceived the primary object as need satisfying and is unable to reach out to the therapist.

28. Blind children need experience with forward and sideways direction, deaf children with sideways and backward direction.

Dance-Movement Therapy Techniques:

Movement activities involving the horizontal direction stressing shaping sideways and across the body.

This is often carried out through the use of location of objects in space. For example, reaching out in a spoke-like manner to grasp an object or a hand. (All categories)

Related elements: Enactive and iconic levels of cognition, space pre-efforts, object-ambivalent or semi-autonomous relationship with the therapist. One-to-one, parallel, or task group.

4. Vertical Directional Shape

A. Maladaptive Behavior: Difficulty in adaptively moving in an arc-like or spoke-like manner in the vertical.

Dance-Movement Therapy Techniques:

Movement activities involving the vertical direction stressing shaping upward and downward. For example, suggest that the group become something, such as, a machine that has up and down moving parts. (All categories)

B. Maladaptive Behavior: Difficulty in maintaining weight constancy.

Dance-Movement Therapy Techniques:

Activities which assist the individual in being aware of and adaptively utilizing his center of gravity.

Here, it is often best not to cloud the difficulty through the use of imagery. For some the sensate experience of getting in touch with how the weight changes from, for example a seated to a standing position is where a therapist could begin. (All categories)

Related elements: Enactive and iconic levels of cognition, object-ambivalent or semi-autonomous relationship; one-to-one, parallel, or task group; use of weight pre-effort.

5. Sagittal Directional Shape

Maladaptive Behavior: Difficulty in adaptively moving in an arc-like or spoke-like manner in the sagittal direction.

Dance-Movement Therapy Techniques:

Movement activities involving the sagittal direction stressing forward and backward patterns.

These can be as simple as moving a circular group into the center and back out again. (All categories)

Related elements: Enactive and iconic levels; object-ambivalent or semi-autonomous relationship; use of time pre-efforts, one-to-one, parallel, or task group.

6. Horizontal Shaping

A. Maladaptive Behavior: Difficulty in adaptively shaping in the horizontal plane by spreading and/or enclosing, such as an individual who continually turns people away with scattering gestures when internally he desperately longs for closeness.

Dance-Movement Therapy Techniques:

1. Movement activities involving general use of spreading and enclosing patterns.

   For example, suggest to a group in a circle that in the center there are all the things they want. Have them gather and verbally identify them and hold them close to themselves. (All categories)

2. Activities which make use of objects to help facilitate the organization of this level.

   Such as the utilization of sheets of material for capes. If it is a children's group, the therapist might suggest that they become birds, butterflies, or even villains and show them how to hold onto the edge of the cape and spread it open and closed such that only their eyes peer out. (All categories)

3. Movement improvisations entailing the archetypal connection to earth mother goddesses such as Demeter and other goddesses who facilitated the sowing of fields and the gathering of the harvest. This experience may be followed by verbal reflection of the seeds of each individual's psychology which are beginning to be planted in their lives along with fantasies of future harvests. (Adult, neurotic)

B. Maladaptive Behavior: Difficulty in adaptively exploring all the possibilities when attending to a situation. For example, someone who can only see his side of a situation.

Dance-Movement Therapy Techniques:

1. Movement activities which involve the exploration of the space around the person (real or imaginary). For example, create an environment which requires the moving of certain objects in space to find a particular object or person. (All categories)

2. Movement improvisations which explore an inner imagined environment such as, a body of water or a wilderness. A suggestion can be offered that there is some object or message for the person somewhere, but he must investigate thoroughly to find it. (Adult, neurotic, adolescent)

   Related elements: Use of spatial efforts, parallel or task group, object-ambivalent, or semi-autonomous relationship with the therapist.

7. Vertical Shaping

   A. Maladaptive Behavior: Difficulty in adaptively shaping in the vertical plane either by rising or sinking. For example, an individual might always "sink" into oblivion when he is asked to "rise" to the occasion as with the meeting of new people or the involvement in novel situations.

   Dance-Movement Therapy Techniques:

   1. Movement activities involving the use of rising and sinking patterns.

      Such as, suggest to a group of children that they are rising in an escalator (have them start in a squat position), or have them pretend to be flowers who are asleep and then rise upward and outward toward the sun (a held light) and then sink back down at nighttime. (All categories with changes of imagery)

   2. Archetypal improvisations which stress interaction between the polarity of "the earth is my Mother, the sky is my Father" (Whitehouse, 1979). (All populations with ego functioning)

   B. Maladaptive Behavior: Difficulty in adaptively presenting himself; for example, someone who has difficulty standing on his own two feet due to low self-esteem.

   Dance-Movement Therapy Techniques:

   Movement activities involving the presentation of self in various situations.

   For example, have a group wander amongst each other and whenever they pass someone suggest to them that they stand up tall and "snub" the person. (All categories)

   Or, the therapist may wish to use imagery; such as, having a person play the proud matador with another being the bull. (All categories)

   Related elements: Use of weight efforts; parallel or task group; object ambivalent or semi-autonomous relationship with the therapist.

8. Sagittal Shaping

   A. Maladaptive Behavior: Difficulty in adaptively shaping in the sagittal plane either through advancing and/or retreating. For example, someone who maintains a retreating pattern for every situation.

   Dance-Movement Therapy Techniques:

   Movement activities involving the use of advancing and retreating.

   For example, suggest to a group of children that they slowly advance toward a haunted house and when they arrive there to quickly retreat. Be sure to have everyone start low and rise as they move forward, reversing the response during the retreat. (All categories)

   B. Maladaptive Behavior: Difficulty in the operation of tasks when adaptively necessary. For example, a man might be able to think out what to do in situations but yet be unable to ever carry out any of his ideas.

   Dance-Movement Therapy Techniques:

   Movement activities involving the carrying out of an activity through various forms of locomotion. For example, have the person anticipate what is to come in a real or imaginary drama and have him act on his decision. If he has a tendency toward acceleration, work on retreating patterns first, with a tendency toward deceleration-advancing patterns.

   Related elements: Use of time efforts, parallel or task group, object ambivalent or semi-autonomous therapeutic relationship.

9. Combination of Two Qualities in Shaping

   Maladaptive Behavior: Difficulty in adaptively combining two qualities in shaping aspects of vertical and horizontal planes, vertical and sagittal planes, or horizontal and sagittal planes.

   Dance-Movement Therapy Techniques:

   Movement activities involving the use of combinations of the various patterns of two shapes in space.

   Such as alternating enclosing and sinking with spreading and rising within the person's own timing. (All categories when age-appropriate)

   Related elements: Use of inner attitude affinities, parallel or task group, semi-autonomous, or chumship relationship.

10. Combination of Three Qualities in Shaping

A. Maladaptive Behavior: Difficulty in adaptively combining three qualities in shaping. For example, an adolescent might have problems in reforming his identity, and may be helped by learning to combine shape qualities in the relating to the environment.

Dance-Movement Therapy Techniques:

Movement activities which involve the combining of three shape qualities in space.

For example, as with the two-shape suggestion, alternate patterns of enclosing, sinking, and retreating with spreading, rising, and advancing toward an object in space. (All categories)

B. Maladaptive Behavior: Difficulty in adaptively shaping in a peripheral, transverse, and/or central pattern. Schizophrenic individuals will quite often lack central or transverse patterning. Their movements are only on the periphery, as many are threatened by involvement of the self with the environment.

Dance-Movement Therapy Techniques:

Movement activities which involve peripheral, transverse, and/or central patterns in shaping.

For example, if an individual has difficulty utilizing more central shaping, the therapist might commence where the individual is most comfortable; i.e., if predominant combination within his repertoire is retreating, sinking, and enclosing, suggest to him that he start the movement in his torso as if hit in the stomach. (All categories with change in imagery)

Related elements: Use of related externalized drives; parallel, task, egocentric, and cooperative group; semi-autonomous, chumship, or autonomous relationship with therapist.

### Interrelationship Between Effort and Shape

Integration of the effort-shape components will be more effective if they are taught jointly. Since each effort has its corresponding shape, both elements will act toward reinforcing each other. If an individual exhibits a preponderance of efforts over shape, he will appear to be aloof; he may possess adequate drives but no ability to direct his need satisfaction to the appropriate object in the environment. He may have a somewhat-functioning ego, but he would be bereft of the capacity to relate to others.

Conversely, if the individual demonstrates far more shaping than efforts, his relationship to his environment will lack feeling and energy; like a "walking zombie," he will move affectlessly through his daily existence.

With regard to the use of efforts: The gain-expense ratio, or the relationship between the amount of flow changes (from free to bound or bound to free) as versus effort attributes (i.e., light, strong, quick, etc.), utilized in each effort component or single movement demonstrates the degree to which affect is differentiated and rigid or spontaneous. For example, two times as many attributes as flow changes within each effort action shows an individual lacking in spontaneity, whereas six times as many flow changes to attributes depicts a child-like personality (Kestenberg).

The load factor (Kestenberg), another concept, measures the complexity of movement in the average amount of effort attributes used in each effort action component. This computation seems to correlate with I.Q. as well as with emotional pathology; 33% would be seen as low, 55% as high.

It should also be noted that a high discrepancy between space efforts and horizontal shaping, weight efforts and vertical shaping, and/or time efforts and sagittal shaping is indicative of conflict behavior (Kestenberg, Lamb). If effort is matched with shape skills in communication, presentation of self and ideas, and the carrying out of one's life, the individual will probably be functioning more adaptively (Lamb). This functioning correspondence also invites interaction with others in the area which is being exhibited (Ramsden). For example, if an individual talking with another utilizes spatial efforts with appropriate horizontal shaping in the communicational sphere, the other person will be more readily able to attend to and receive a clear message, thus facilitating his response. If on the other hand, using directness, he continuously tilts his torso forward and back, gesturing in the vertical plane, the other may feel that he is not that interested or involved in truly sharing with him what he feels nor interested in his response. The other person has picked up a certain inconsistency in the individual's behavior, thus what is responded to often becomes unclear. (See outline for movement profile in the appendix for a more depth view of tension and shape flow, efforts and shape, intra- and intersystemic relationships.)

| EFFORT | SHAPE |
|---|---|
| *Tension Flow* | *Shape Flow Design* |
| Flow adjustment | Looping, undulent |
| Even intensity | Linear |
| Low intensity | Low amplitude |
| High intensity | High amplitude |
| Gradual increase in intensity | Soft reversal |
| Steep increase in intensity | Angular reversal |

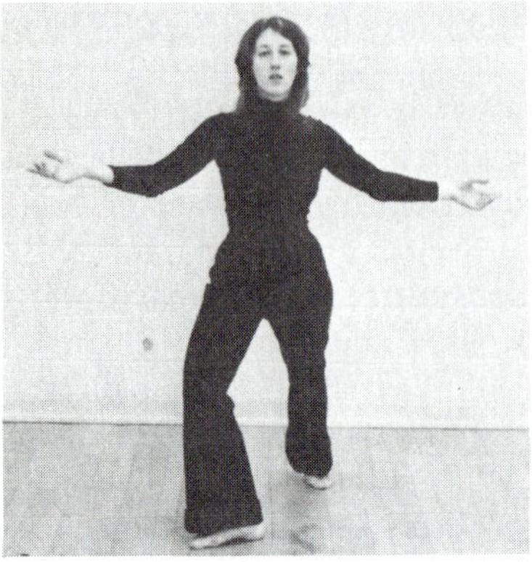

Widening

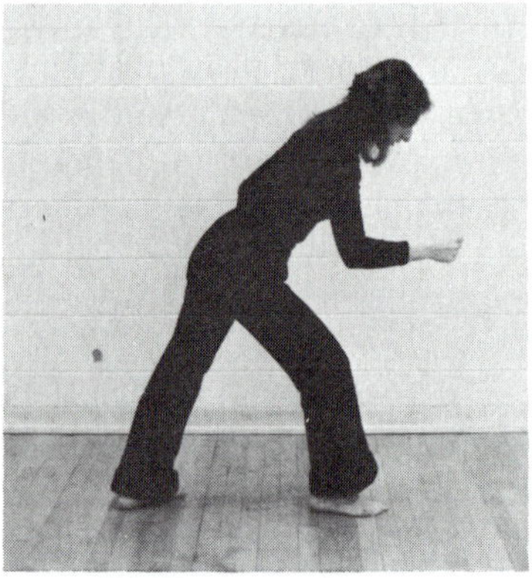

Enclosing

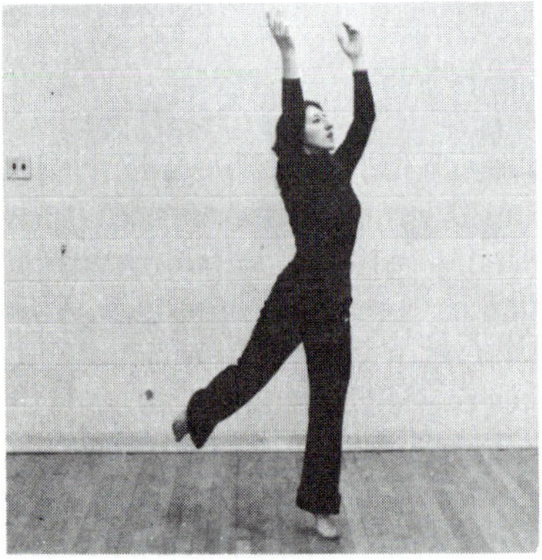

Ascending

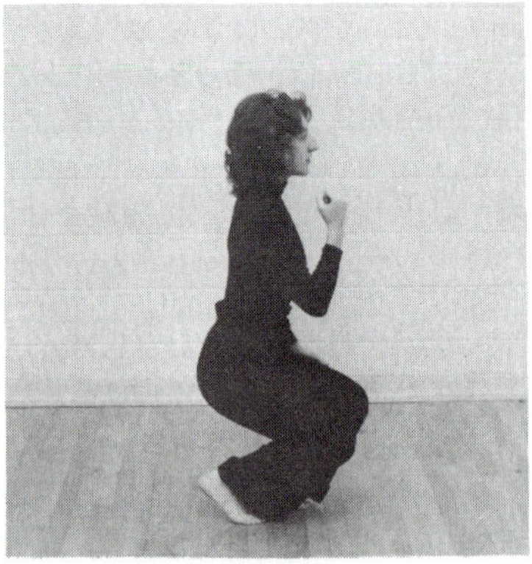

Descending

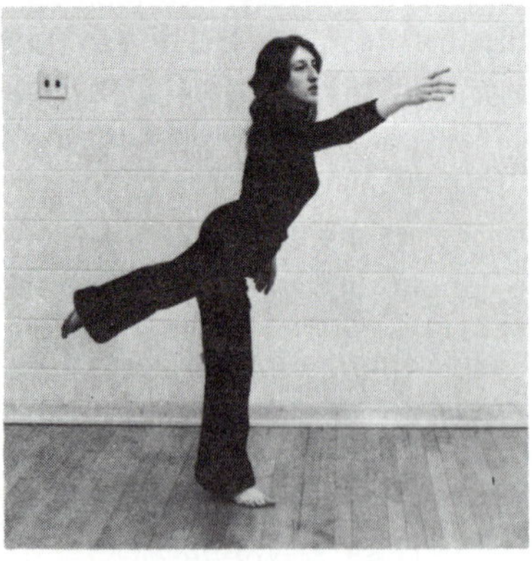

Advancing

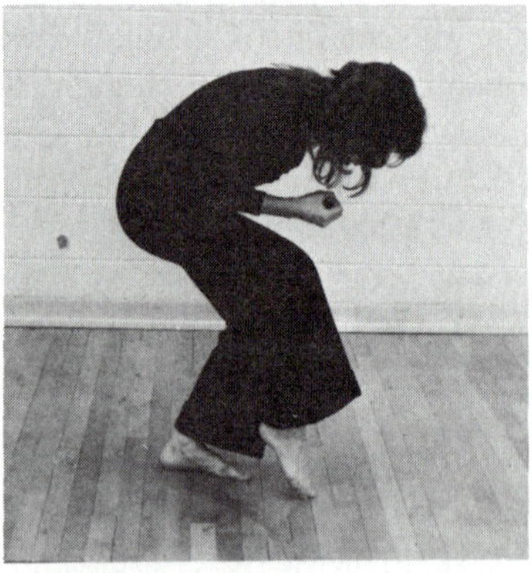

Retreating

**Figure III.5.** Shaping

| | |
|---|---|
| *Pre-effort* | *Directional Shape* |
| Flexible | Sideways |
| Channeled | Across the body |
| Gentle | Upward |
| Vehement | Downward |
| Hesitation | Backward |
| *Effort* | *Shaping* |
| Indirect | Spreading |
| Direct | Enclosing |
| Light | Ascending |
| Strong | Descending |
| Deceleration | Advancing |
| Acceleration | Retreating |

FLOW

| | |
|---|---|
| *Tension Flow* | *Shape Flow* |
| Free | Growing |
| Bound | Shrinking |

## POSTURE-GESTURE LEVELS OF ORGANIZATION

Among the behavioral phenomena which may be utilized as indicators of developmental adaptive organization in movement, are the uses of posture and gesture. These two concepts were developed by Warren Lamb and have been enlarged upon in his work as a management consultant.

Gesture is defined simply as action which is confined to one or more parts of the body without encompassing the whole body.

Posture is action involving a continuous adjustment of every part of the body with consistency in the process of variation.[29] When this occurs, the motion possesses a coordination of flow or tone throughout.

Clearly both postural and gestural movements are needed to adequately adapt to the environment. Although observations of individual posture-gesture patterns demonstrate that there are idiosyncratic ranges, it is generally felt that the more a person can enlarge his repertoire, especially where posture and gesture are seen to overlap, the more he is said to be acting in accordance with his real self.[30]

29. Warren Lamb, *Posture and Gesture* (London: Gerald Duckworth & Co., 1965), p. 16.

30. *Ibid.*, p. 85. It is important to note here that within certain contexts naturally gesture is more appropriate than a G-P or P-G merger. For example, for a Dance-Movement Therapist to utilize a P-G merger when greeting a schizophrenic individual for the first time would be quite inappropriate. (A schizophrenic generally moves using only peripheral gestures. If the therapist greeted him with a postural movement, he would not be meeting the person at his level of communication.)

Generally, gestural efforts relate to an individual's capabilities, and gestural shapes with his self-appraisal. Postural efforts and shapes reflect superego functioning. Postural efforts relate to expressions from the punitive superego and address adaptation to forbidden or permissible actions; while shaping in postures reflects the individual's aspirations, ego ideal, and/or denigrations of self in relation to other objects (Kestenberg, 1980).

Based on the study of current findings, Christensen formulated some propositions concerning the importance of postural movement. Among them are the following:

1. The release of basis organismic response presupposes a postural basis.
2. Their release can be interfered with by a dissolution of their postural basis, and
3. The permanent dissolution of the postural basis for an organismic response will have repercussions on the organism's breathing pattern (Page 75).

Thus in order for motoric behavior utilized in emotional expression and basic need gratification to be fully organized and integrated, it must involve a full postural merger with the appropriate flow of breath.

### Posture-Gesture Levels of Organization

1. Posture-Gesture Flow

   This involves the capacity for tension and shape flow variation utilizing both postural and gestural movement.

2. Merging of Gesture Systems

   The merging of gesture systems involves the ability to link any effort or shape quality with another so that one attribute merges into another within a gestural sequence.[31]

3. Merging of Posture-Gesture Systems

   The merging of P-G systems involves the ability to link posture with gesture while maintaining consistent shaping and/or efforts. Gestural shaping and/or efforts may be "backed up" by postural movement which are consistent in quality with the gesture, or posture may be "carried on" by gesture (Lamb).[32] In either case one must

31. For example, an arm raised upwards in a light upbeat flowing into an arc-like forward quick, direct motion.

32. Lamb, *op. cit.*, p. 37.

evolve and flow from the other. All attributes of effort (i.e., those adapting to space, weight, and time) as well as those qualities of shape, must be able to be utilized in posture-gesture merging in order for this level to be fully organized.

### Related Maladaptive Behavior with Suggested Methods and Techniques for Dance-Movement Therapy

1. Posture-Gesture Flow

   A. Maladaptive Behavior: The difficulty in adaptively varying tension and/or shape flow with postural movements; for example, an individual might be suppressing sexual drive due to guilt or anxiety which manifests itself in a blocked pelvic area.

   Dance-Movement Therapy Techniques:

   Movement activities which involve the use of tension and/or shape flow with postural movements. For example, the therapist might first ascertain which aspects of flow a woman prefers within her gestural repertoire. She might, for example, move a great deal utilizing the adjustment of tension flow with a corresponding undulent, looping quality in shape flow. The therapist could then suggest to her to allow the gestural quality to flow throughout her body. (All categories)

   B. Maladaptive Behavior: The difficulty in adaptively merging posture with gesture in tension and/or shape flow. This could show itself in a tense individual who has been unable to merge his gestural strivings into postural adjustment.

   Dance-Movement Therapy Techniques:

   1. Movement activity encompassing changes of flow involving evolution from gestural to postural patterns and from postural to gestural. For example, a pattern which makes use of breathing as a rhythmic force in the flow of gestural (the chest and diaphragm) to postural (the whole body) movement.
   2. Movement activities which involve asymmetrical or unipolar shape flow; for example, the person initially responds asymmetrically in a gesture to a stimulus. This may take the form of an initial unipolar widening or or narrowing, lengthening or shortening, and/or bulging or hollowing followed successively by the whole body. (All categories)

      Related elements: One-to-one or parallel group. Egocentric, or object ambivalent relationship with therapist.

2. Merging of Gesture Systems

Maladaptive Behavior: Difficulty in adaptively merging gesture systems in effort and/or shape. Autistic children often have bizarre unrelated gestures involving ritualistic repetitive mannerisms.

Dance-Movement Therapy Techniques:

Movement patterns involving the linking of various effort attributes of space, weight, and time and/or shape attributes of communication, presentation, and operation, as well as the combination of effort-shape affinities in merging gestural systems.

Here again, the therapist may wish to make use of the person's preferred efforts and/or shapes. It also is of help to make use of related tension and/or shape flow attributes to evolve the person into the corresponding efforts and/or shapes which entail more ego adaptation:

| *Tension Flow* | evolve to | *Effort* |
|---|---|---|
| Flow adjustment | " | indirectness |
| Even intensity | " | directness |
| Low intensity | " | lightness |
| High intensity | " | strength |
| Gradual increase in intensity | " | slowness |
| Steep increase in intensity | " | quickness |
| *Shape Flow Design* | evolve to | *Shaping* |
| Looping, undulent | " | spreading |
| Linear | " | enclosing |
| Low amplitude | " | ascending |
| High amplitude | " | descending |
| Soft reversal | " | advancing |
| Angular reversal | " | retreating |
| (All categories) | | |

Related elements: One-to-one, or parallel group, object-ambivalent or semi-autonomous relationship with therapist.

3. Merging of Posture-Gesture Systems

   A. Maladaptive Behavior: Difficulty in adaptively linking gesture with posture and/or posture with gesture while maintaining any consistent shaping and/or efforts. A person in which P-G merger was not present might take on a doll-like or puppet-like quality in his movement.[33] His repertoire would have an artificial quality due to the lack of postural adjustment.

33. Lamb, *ibid.*, pp. 31–32.

Dance-Movement Therapy Techniques:

1. Movement patterns which involve the linking of a posture with a gesture or vice versa while maintaining consistent shaping and/or efforts.

   Such as:

   Posture-gesture merging activities which have indirect application to daily tasks with which the individual or individuals have difficulty.

   For example:

   1. Analyze the appropriate effort-shape P-G merging for a key point in a daily task of the individual.
   2. Have the individual fully integrate this pattern so that his original limited movement (usually solely gestural in nature) is extended.
   3. Have the individual apply this pattern to the appropriate activity or activities.[34] (Adults, individuals, neurotics)
2. Movement activities which utilize real or imaginary sports activities which stress P-G mergers, such as the pitching of a baseball. (All categories)

B. Maladaptive Behavior: Extraneous movement patterns utilized in lieu of a natural signature of posture-gesture overlap.[35] For example, if an individual had much unmerged posture, it might demonstrate "a lack of cultivation, either skill training, education generally, or social development,"[36] or it may reflect a superego which can't come to agreement with the ego's mediation of id impulses.

Dance-Movement Therapy Techniques:

1. The therapist should not expect to change the above example's way of handling or ordering his physical behavior, if this pattern is due to his personal style of responding to "a lack of cultivation" in a particular area. What can be done is to increase the client's ability in the area in question in terms of the particular movement repertoire needed to perform the task. If it is a job situation, the therapist might wish to advise the person

34. *Ibid.*, p. 171.
35. *Ibid.*, p. 66.
36. *Ibid.*

if his own repertoire is not compatible with what is required. (All categories except children)

2. Movement improvisations which explore the movement and associated stance of the superego as one polarity and the stance of the id-ego gesture as the other. Encourage the individual to take on both personifications, having them relate to each other and see if a middle ground or merger can be made through resolution of the conflict. (All categories)

C. Maladaptive Behavior: Minimal or no adaptive exhibition of emotions on a postural level. This could be the type of person whose so-called expressions of emotion are not really believable. For example, a woman greets a lover by extending her arms as if to embrace, but when he moves toward her she maintains her torso in a rigid tense manner.

Dance-Movement Therapy Techniques:

1. Movement which involves taking an emotion, expressing it gesturally, and evolving it into a postural form (the more postural an expression of emotion, the more meaningful it is to the individual).

   For example, the therapist might start the pattern utilizing the portion of the body most often used in gestures by that person or group (generally the hands and forearms), and evolve them into an expressive pattern such as strong, quick, indirect-slashes moving first the arms, then shoulders, upper torso, etc. (All categories)

2. Movement activities in which verbalization is incorporated into the pattern "verbal communication backed up by consistent postural movement will be experienced as a convincing and sincere expression of the verbal message."[37]

   For example, an individual who is involved with stamping (strong, quick, direct) his leg while merging in repeated vertical postures might yell each time, "I won't!" (All categories)

   Related elements: Parallel, task, or egocentric-cooperative group; semi-autonomous or chumship relationship with therapist.

37. Portion of study carried out by Warren Lamb Associates and presented at the 1971 Dance Notation Bureau Conference in New York.

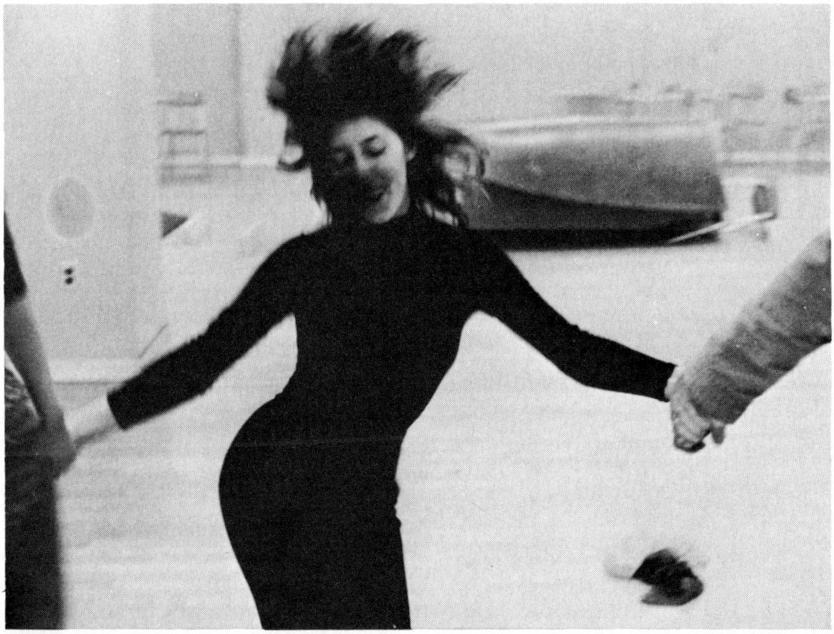

Merger of posture-gesture flow

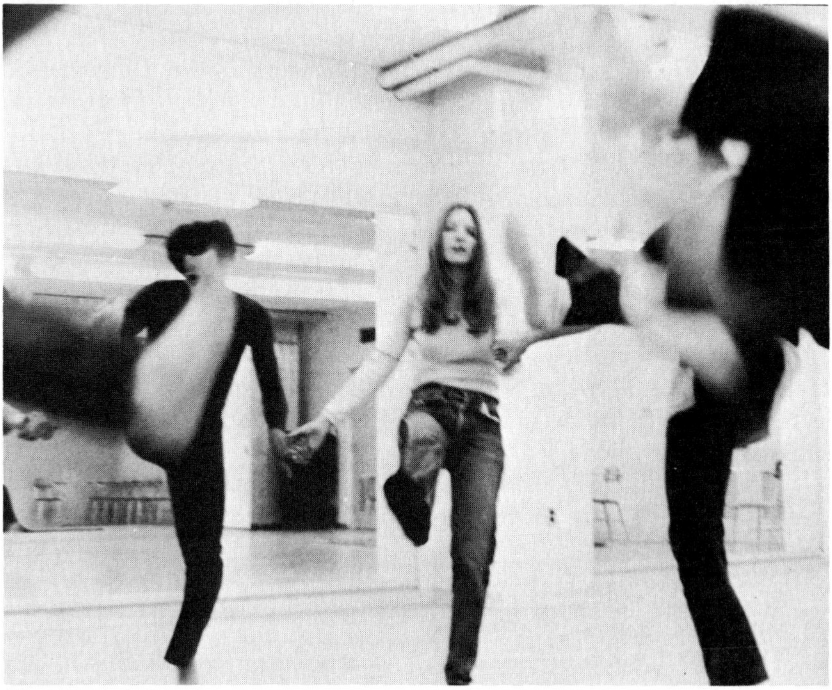

Merger of E/S gesture systems

## TENSION FLOW RHYTHMS LEVELS OF ORGANIZATION

The importance of the role of rhythm in human development and in the learning of adaptive patterns has generally been acknowledged among both psychologists and educators. Psychotherapists have also observed that rhythm is one of the few basic qualities that is pleasurable to a regressed individual; it is therefore often one of the few avenues of communication open to the therapist. Kestenberg, restating Kris says, "the primitive rhythm of affective discharge as it is modified by the ego becomes a vehicle for non-verbal communication."[38]

Rhythm is one element which is generally present in a Dance-Movement Therapy session; therapists make use of it but quite often only on a superficial basis. Because of its importance to the individual and therefore to the therapeutic process, this tool cannot be overlooked or casually used. Rhythm is especially significant if the individual's primary or *only* method of communication is on a non-verbal level. Rhythm, because of its major importance, then becomes the basic medium for interaction and therapy. Psychiatrists, psychologists, and other psychotherapists (unless they have studied Dance Therapy) do not have facility with this tool. The knowledgeable movement therapist has, however, and can therefore serve a primary role in the psychotherapy of an individual who could not be engaged in therapy using more traditional methods.

This primitive method of communication acts also to integrate the total being. It has been found that when the flow of rhythm involves all the muscle systems, an increased awareness of the total body and a sense of well being quite often ensue.

However, a therapist who superimposes his own natural rhythmic pattern or tires to use an alien beat found in some piece of music, rather than first observing the rhythmic level of his client, may produce a negative reaction and serve to further withdraw an already regressed individual.

The rhythms that will be discussed here are those described by Dr. Judith Kestenberg. She states:

"Rhythms of tension flow serve need satisfaction such as sucking, defecating, or urinating. With the onset of psychic functioning the tension flow apparatus is used for drive discharge in such a way that oral, anal, urethal, and genital drives find their expression in appropriate motor rhythms."[39]

True differentiation and organization are contingent upon these motor channels being established at the appropriate discharge zone.

38. Judith Kestenberg, M.D., "The Role of Movement Patterns in Development: I. Rhythms of Movement," *Psychoanalytic Quarterly,* XXXIV (1965), p. 3.

39. Judith Kestenberg, H. Marcus, E. Robbins, J. Berlowe, and A. Buelte, "Development of a Young Child as Expressed Through Bodily Movement," unprinted paper. Sands Point, New York, p. 4. It is also important to note here that "Rhythms in shape flow give structure to the changes of tension by providing patterns of interaction with need-satisfying or frustrating stimuli and objects," p. 4.

| Tension FLow Rhythm | Need | Motoric Drive Discharge | Discharge Zone |
|---|---|---|---|
| Oral libidinal | Nourishment | Sucking | Mouth |
| Oral Aggressive | Nourishment | Biting (teething) Chewing | Mouth |
| Anal Libidinal | Elimination Defecation | Expelling, twisting | Anal sphincter |
| Anal Sadistic | Elimination Defecation | Shaping evacuation control Straining, holding, expelling | Anal sphincter |
| Urethral Libidinal | Elimination Micturition | Flowing, urinating | Bladder, urethra |
| Urethral Sadistic | Elimination Micturition | Bladder control Running, darting, Stopping | Bladder, urethra |
| Inner Genital | Sexual gratification | Embracing, inclusive floating | Genitals |
| Phallic (outer Genital) | Sexual gratification | Introducing, ballistic leaping, jumping | Genitals |
| Genital | Sexual gratification | Adult orgasm | Genitals |

When drive discharge is localized, the ego is then able to control and mediate the drive.

These rhythms exist in pure and mixed form in combination with each other. All rhythms when organized should be present in pure form for adaptive functioning. An integrated adult will have an increased ratio of mixed rhythms to pure (5:1), denoting a higher degree of sublimation, as well as more libidinal rhythms than sadistic in mixed form stressing subtleties of indulging pleasurable need gratification over aggressive-sadistic discharge (Kestenberg).

### Tension Flow Rhythms Levels of Organization[40]

1. Oral Libidinal

   This level involves the ability to control libidnal oral rhythms of tension flow which aids in the development of a primary object relationship. This phase is inclusive of Mahler's (1968) stages of normal autism, symbiosis which peeks at around five months and beginning differentiation in which the sensori perspective stance of the infant serves body boundary delineation. The oral rhythm can be described as smooth, repetitive undulations from free to bound flow which is characterized by sucking. 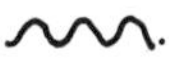. The primary zone

40. Adapted from Kestenberg, ibid.

for this movement is, of course, the mouth; however, if an infant is viewed during normal breast feeding the observer will note that the oral rhythm may be carried throughout the body. In order for the infant to organize this task he must perceive his initial experience with the environment (via his mouth) as a pleasant and need-satisfying one. It is vital, therefore, that the mother (his first environment) appropriately mediate his sucking rhythms, neither bulging her breast so that the infant's control over nursing is totally curtailed, nor withdrawing it out of anger or fear of rejection. Mother's body must be soft and somewhat yielding to provide an indulging cushion of tender acceptance. A body that is bound or flaccid-limp will transmit negative kinesthetic cues and promote an atmosphere of potential anxiety and mistrust. Attunement to the oral rhythm promotes and encourages the symbiotic relationship.[41]

2. Oral Aggressive

This involves the ability to control oral sadistic rhythms of tension flow which serve to aid in the further evolution of differentiation of the individual from his environment.

The oral aggressive rhythm can be defined as jerky, sharp, repetitive fluctuations from free to bound flow. This is the rythm of biting and chewing. 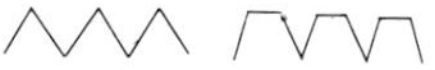 . The rhythm is first observed in teething when the infant attempts to work his milk teeth through his gums. As with oral incorporative rhythms, these rhythms may be found in other areas of the body—particularly in the reaching out for and grasping and releasing of objects.

3. Anal Libidinal

This involves the ability to control anal libidinal rhythms of tension flow which aid in the adjustment to new positions and trial actions. There is a playful quality to this rhythm reflecting a delicate refinement of feeling and a willingness to change.

This rhythm is characterized as having predominantly low tension with small changes in intensity. 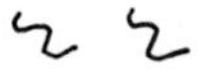 .

Here the ability to coordinate breathing with defecation as well as to integrate and experience the "letting go modality" as part of the personality are vital (Christensen). This separation-individuation process encompasses much of the practicing subphase in which the child checks and rechecks mother's presence (Mahler).

41. Exaggerated attunement fosters fears of engulfment. Its reverse, exaggerated clashing of rhythms, fosters separation fears. (Kestenberg)

4. Anal Sadistic

This involves the ability to control anal sadistic flow patterns which further serve in presentation and confrontation as well as the awareness of qualities of weight. Independence and more of a sense of autonomy evolves here in the so-called "terrible two's." The rapprochement subphase of object relationship development is in operation during the dominence of this rhythm. Here the child basks in his productions and wishes mother to share and acknowledge every experience. Mother continues to be split into good or bad object (Mahler).

This rhythm is defined as having a high intensity of even bound flow with eventual relaxation into a free flow state

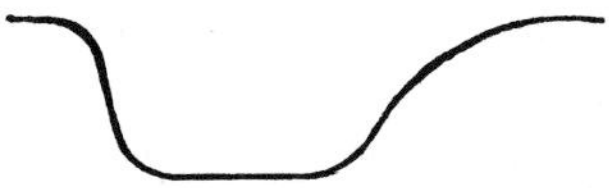

The individual must be able to "maintain high tension while squatting (shortening of body shape) and to lengthen in low tension."[42] Bowel control is present here as well as movements of a holding expelling quality in other parts of the body. The rhythm reflects the ability to hold back and persist with caution.

5. Urethral Libidinal

This involves the ability to control urethral libidinal rhythmic tension flow patterns which serve in the operation of tasks and decisions. This is a passive level in which the toddler flows everywhere with limitless time. The developmental task entails the capacity to experience the pleasure of letting go. Body boundaries become liquid. Toddlers use mother's solid body to reinstate a sense of body delineation.

This rhythm is characterized by gradual decrease and increase intension

6. Urethral Sadistic

This involves the ability to control urethral sadistic rhythmic tension flow patterns which serve in the mastery of locomotion and in the capacity to start and stop suddenly. The developmental physiologic task is that of bladder control.

42. Kestenberg, *op. cit.* p. 16

This rhythm is defined as having sharp reversals from free to bound flow, often starting and stopping suddenly.

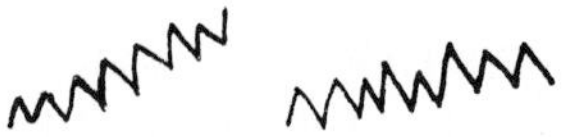

7. Inner Genital Libidinal

This involves the capacity to control inner genital libidinal patterns which serve to aid in the development of receptivity. Inclusive, indulging behavior, as well as identification with mother or surrogate figure are part of this level of organization. The inner genital rhythm entails the realm of inner sensations, i.e., the spreading of genital excitement inside the body. For females the discharge zone is the vagina and uterus; for males, the prostate and vas deferens. Important to note here is that this internal rhythm is subject to more primary process than secondary process expression, and in adult years its presence in men reflects their level of integration of their anima (their relationship to their internal feminine).

This rhythm is characterized by undulant wavy flat transitions between free and bound flow.

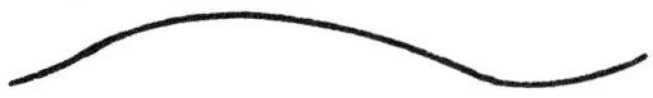

8. Inner Genital Sadistic

This involves the ability to control inner genital sadistic rhythmic flow which serves to aid in the development of orgiastic states and during childbirth.

This rhythm is characterized by large undulant transitions between free and bound flow.

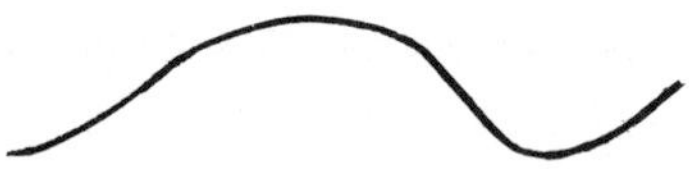

9. Phallic Libidinal (Outer Genital Libidinal)

This involves the ability to control external genital libidinal rhythms and is characterized by high intensity rounded flow adjustments with steep increases and decreases in tension. Masturbatory activities are seen at this stage, the focuses of which are the penis for males and the clitoris for females.

Intrusive behavior, as well as identification with father or surrogate figure are part of this level of organization. Also inclusive in the developmental task of this phase is the differentiation between action thinking and word thinking. For women, its presence and integration reflects their level of individuation of their animus (their relationship to their internal masculine).

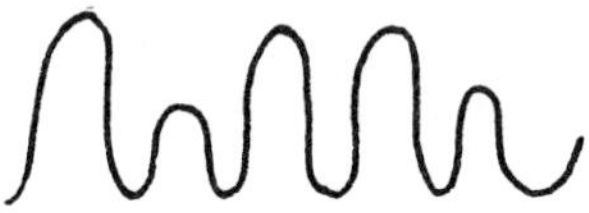

10. Phallic Sadistic (Outer Genital Sadistic)

This involves the ability to control external genital aggressive rhythms which characterize leaps and the ballistic qualities in most sports activities. Impulses from internal sex organs are externalized.

It is characterized by high intensity sharp flow adjustment with steep increases and decreases in tension.

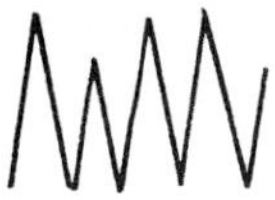

11. Genital Rhythm

This involves the ability to combine and control outer and inner genital rhythms. This P-F rhythm,[43] as it has been named by Marcus and Kestenberg, is the predominating characteristic genital rhythm of normal adults, and is exhibited during coitus and full-body orgasm.

It is characterized by medium-intensity transitions.

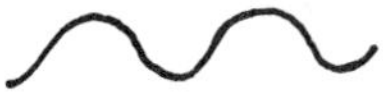

## Related Maladaptive Behavior with Suggested Methods and Techniques for Dance-Movement Therapy

1. Oral Libidinal

A. Maladaptive Behavior: Difficulty in the utilization of a pure oral libidinal rhythm[44] when adaptively appropriate. An individual might be unable to comfort himself during a sad experience by, for ex-

43. Phallic-feminine rhythm

44. Pure rhythms are: oral, oral aggressive, anal, anal sadistic, urethral, urethral aggressive, inner genital, inner genital sadistic, outer genital, outer genital sadistic, sadistic. Examples of mixed rhythms: oral-anal, oral sadistic-phallic, inner genital-inner genital sadistic, etc. The presence of rhythms in a pure form is adaptively needed in a functioning individual. A normal adult will have mixed rhythms; however, if rhythms in their pure form are not present, needed drive investment and differentiation will not occur. (Kestenberg)

ample, a rocking pattern or a gesture involving the stroking of the face or the opposite arm due to early severe narcissistic wounds. On a more pathological level there may be a regression or fixation to the autistic phase in which deanimation, dedifferentiation, and an inability to respond to the buffering oral rhythms of the primary object results (Mahler, 1968).

Dance-Movement Therapy Techniques:

1. Movement activities involving the control of smooth, repetitive undulations from free to bound flow and from growing to shrinking in shaping. It is generally easiest if the movement evolves from gesture and links onto posture. For example, involve the person in a rocking pattern, first holding the person's hand and moving it in a rocking fashion with gradual involvement of the torso and whole body. If the person is seated the therapist may utilize a sagittal rocking pattern to slowly rock him to a standing position. Taking both hands, the clinician may gently sway with the person to the beat of music which reinforces this rhythmic pattern. (All categories especially schizophrenia, childhood psychosis, and those suffering from withdrawal reactions)
2. Movement activities involving passive manipulation of the individual by the therapist in an oral rhythm, such as the rocking of an individual. (Psychotics, children, individuals, some individuals with personality disorders.) (See Figure III.6.)

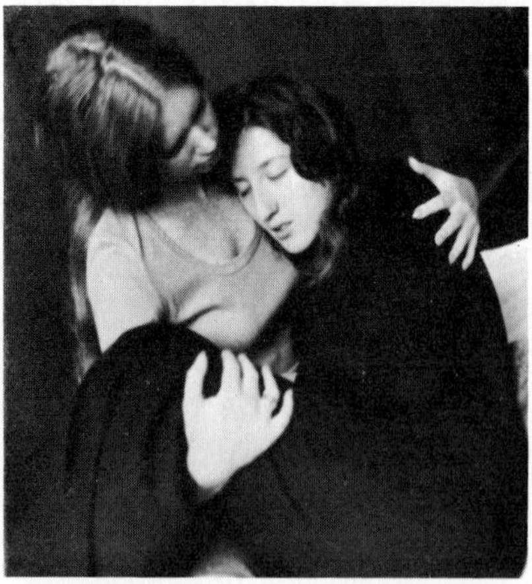

**Figure III.6.** Rocking

3. Movement activities involving taking in and receiving, such as the real or imaginary taking in of a favorite food (suggestion of sweet foods and fruits might be helpful). (All categories)
4. Movement activities involving patting and/or rubbing, such as having each person pat-tap his whole body with an even repetitive motion. (All categories)
5. Movement activities which enlarge upon grasp and release patterns. Such as a G-P merger starting with the opening and closing of the hands ending in a grasp (shrinking, bound flow) release (growing, free flow) pattern involving the whole body. (All categories)
6. Use of verbalizations during session. For example, suggest to the individual or group to repeat "yes" with each oral rhythm, or ask the group to respond to such questions as "What is your favorite sweet?" (All categories)

B. Maladaptive Behavior: Oral Syndrome: bound deep neck muscles and upper back, torso arched, stiffening and resistance of arm and leg extension, tense jaw (Lowen), due to a mother whose empathy was faulty or absent, who did not provide tension relieving gratification, and/or whose body posture and movement was not properly attuned to the infant's needs.

Dance-Movement Therapy Techniques:

Movement activities involving getting in touch with the repressed conflicted oral needs through, free associational movement dramas in which the individual relives traumatic maladaptive infant experiences. Movement explorations which remobilize wishes for parental approval may follow as the therapist encourages "acting in" narcissistic fantasies. As the idealizing transference is strengthened through the movement therapist's unconditional acceptance of the client's "body-mind-self", a "host of meaningful memories" are internalized; and the individual is able to utilize the positive object relationship toward the establishment of a realistic ego ideal (Kohut, 1971, p. 98). (Narcissistic personality disorders)

Related elements: horizontal directional shape, spacial pre-efforts; egocentric relationship with therapist; one-to-one or parallel group; flow of breath; weaning ritual process.

2. Oral Aggressive

A. Maladaptive Behavior: Difficulty adaptively initiating and cessating oral aggressive rhythms. Such as an individual who has difficulty expressing aggression even in its most primitive form.

Dance-Movement Therapy Techniques:

1. Movement activities involving the control of jerky, sharp, repetitive undulations from free to bound flow and from growing to shrinking in shape flow. Such as a dance which emphasizes the maintaining of an accented repetitive beat either by banging the floor with hands or feet, clapping, or use of percussion instruments such as sticks, cymbols, drum. (All categories)
2. Movement activities which facilitate the development of the body ego in which the individual is encouraged to tense and release body parts. This aids in the differentiation of the body from the environment. (All categories)
3. Movement activities which involve seizing and grasping. For example, have each person seize imaginary desired objects such as people, food, love, etc., in the middle of the circle, keeping all of it in their arms. Then each go around to others and try to grasp what they have. (Mutual sharing can also occur here although not component-related.) (All categories)

B. Maladaptive Behavior: An individual with a "hanging on bite" exhibited by a tense throat and jaw and chest, as well as fixed, bound, glaring eyes. The person may be ambitious and rivalrous and literally spit with anger, or he may be unable to yell out at all.

Dance-Movement Therapy Techniques:

1. Use of movement-imagery which facilitates snarling and biting; such as the group all being angry lions or cannibals or on a deeper level through thematic authentic movement suggestions may be made to allow themselves to go into their primordial swamp and image and then embody their swamp creature. (All categories except psychotic)
2. Movement activities involving the exaggeration of the tension in the jaw to facilitate relaxation. Such as having an individual bite onto a towel or food which requires chewing. (Neurotics)

   A reciprocal grab the towel of tug of war is also successful. (All categories) Use of yelling and other verbalizations which help the individual toward differentiation and individualization, such as asking the patient, "I am me; who are you?" (Chace) A group yell is also helpful and it is often more safe. The group may start with a gentle tone and work up to a roar. (All categories)

Related elements: Horizontal direction, and spacial pre-efforts, one-to-one or parallel group; object dependent relationship with therapist; Body-Image: differentiation of the body from the environment

3. Anal Libidinal

A. Maladaptive Behavior: Difficulty in adaptively utilizing anal libidinal rhythms. This could characterize an individual who is excessively involved or fixated at the oral aggressive level; i.e., someone who snaps and "bites" at his environment being unable to respond in a more gentle, playful manner.

Dance-Movement Therapy Techniques:

1. Movement activities involving rhythmic control of low tension with small changes in intensity. Such as use of playful games like peek-a-boo or pat-a-cake with the feet. (Children, groups, individuals, psychotics)
2. Movement which entails brief intervals of holding and releasing, or activities involving brief growing out into space and releasing, such as is found in many ball games. (All categories)
3. Use of ambivalent verbalizations such as "I will, I won't." (All categories)

B. Maladaptive Behavior: Ambivalent, careless, and frustrated individual characterized by an inability to feel committed, often observed moving from leg to leg. In children this often takes the form of constant kicking and slapping; excrements come to be used as ammunition. This behavior can be caused by "a lack of consideration for the child's rhythm, lack of understanding of his feeling of belonging to his own product" (Christensen). In adults the constant need to seek approval reflects poor self feeling the origins of which stem from a paucity of maternal interest and elation in the child's body and his experiences (Mahler).

Dance-Movement Therapy Techniques:

1. Use of props or imagery which can involve messing and smearing. Such as an imaginary walk in mud or "foot-finger painting" while dancing. (All categories except, of course, those who have dirtphobias.)

2. Movement activities which encourage the individual's spontaneous improvisations with strong positive interest and regard for the client's experience and product. (All categories)

   Related elements: Object ambivalent relationship with therapist, parallel group, use of weight pre-efforts and veritcal shape.

4. Anal Sadistic

   A. Maladaptive Behavior: Difficulty in adaptively utilizing anal sadistic rhythms. This can characterize an individual who has a great deal of difficulty standing up for himself, presenting himself in a situation. He may not be able to confront another or to refuse to carry out an offensive order. He may not be able to view individuals as both good and bad simultaneously.

   Dance-Movement Therapy Techniques:

   1. Movement activities involving the rhythmic control of high Intensity even bound flow followed by relaxation into a free flow state both in posture and gesture. For example, suggest to the individual to move to a vertical position from lying supine and/or prone, or have him move from a seated to a standing position using this rhythmic pattern. (All categories)
   2. Movements involving presentation of self as dominant and proud, such as being "the boss" or a peacock. (All categories)
   3. Use of negative verbalizations such as "No," "I won't." (All categories)
   4. Movements involving taking "No" throughout the body. Suggest, "How many ways can you make your body say 'No'?"—e.g., stamp feet, shake your head, etc. (All categories)
   5. Suggest to the patient that he lie on a couch or bed and have him alternately kick his feet and arms while shouting "No!" After a period of time, his head should automatically move from side to side. Any holding back on the part of the patient will be demonstrated by lack of coordination (Lowen). (See Figure III.7.) (Neurotics, adults)
   6. Movements involving imaginary throwing, dropping, destroying, shoving, pushing, and wringing. For example, ask the whole group (or individual) to lift a heavy negative imaginary object in the center of the circle. After they have done this, have them throw it away, stamp on it, or whatever they wish. (All categories)

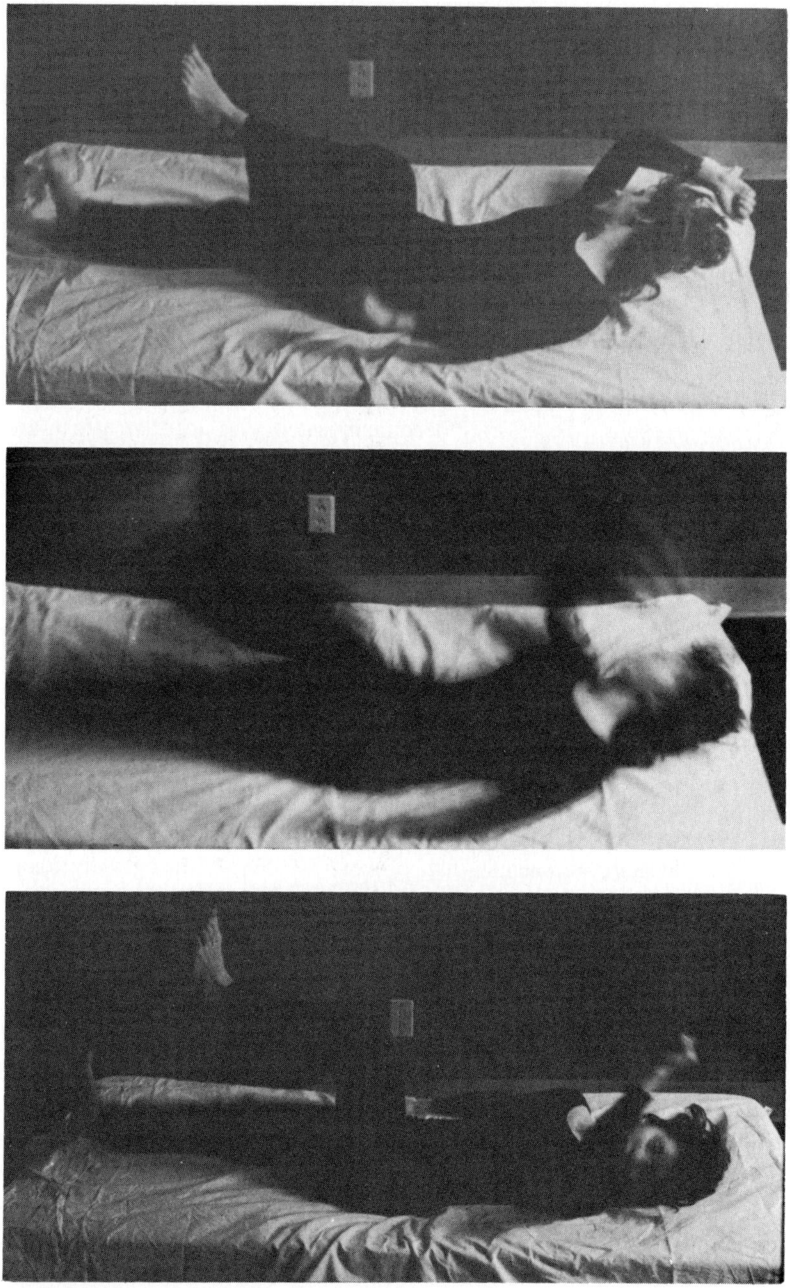

**Figure III.7.** Talking "No" through the body

B. Maladaptive Behavior: Difficulty in completing anal sadistic pattern or a straining inward. This is the individual who some call the "tight-ass" and, by the way, he actually does have a clenched contracted buttocks and tense anal sphincter; his thighs and calves, too, will be bound. With a forward, upward presentational pelvic tilt and a tightening of the shoulders, the characteristic low backache syndrome appears. He may be compulsively meticulous, perfectionistically productive, hostile, and determined, but generally he will have a great deal of difficulty expressing anger, keeping it locked up inside a tense body structure. This behavioral complex may be due to premature parental pressure for bowel control and orderliness and/or to authority figures never allowing the toddler any independent negative response. Feces often become invested with negative affect, and the individual feels himself to literally be a "piece of shit"—one who must keep those "shitty feelings" constipated, bound up inside at all costs.

Dance-Movement Therapy Techniques:

1. Movement activities which stress the vertical, downward release of tension. For example, have the individual arch the upper part of his back over a grounded stool while he is holding on. The person is instructed to push down from this somewhat horizontal position to a vertical one while exhaling with possible vocalization. The finished position is a vertical squat. (See Figure III.8 for more detailed description.) This pattern is then repeated. (Adults, neurotics)

   Related elements: Use of vertical shape and gravitational-weight pre-efforts and efforts, drive-object: investment of aggressive drive in external objects, semi-autonomous relationship with therapist. Parallel group, vestibular perception.

5. Urethral Libidinal

   Maladaptive Behavior: Difficulty in adaptively utilizing urethral libidinal rhythms. This could be shown in an individual who has difficulty allowing himself to move with a relaxed flowing quality, i.e., his movements are always stiff and/or jerky. He is unable to take time to linger on a subject or a person: dawdling and day-dreaming are definitely out of the question. The etiology of this behavior could stem from a family situation which would curtail the pleasurable flow of an idling child with continuous demands for premature bladder control and/or for temporal structure on his carrying out of activities.

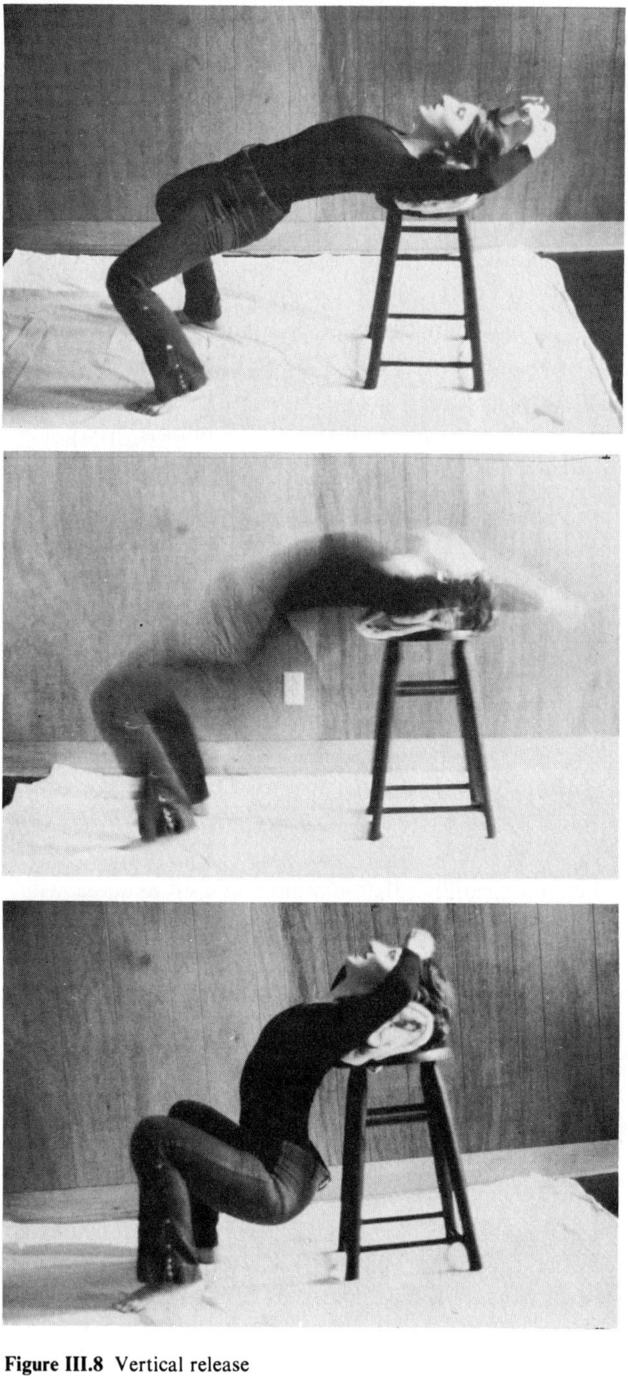

**Figure III.8** Vertical release

Dance-Movement Therapy Techniques:

1. Movement activities involving rhythmic control of gradual decrease and increase in tension with soft reversals in shape flow. For example, dancing to liquid zen meditation music. (All categories)
2. Use of imagery of a derivative of urethral libidinal patterns. For example, being a melting snowman (children) or other forms which involve liquid, or wandering through an imaginary environment. (All categories)
3. Movement activities in liquid environments; such as, heated pools, jacuzzis, hot tubs. (All categories)

   Related elements: Sagittal shape and time efforts, semi-autonomous relationship with therapist, parallel or task group.

6. Urethral Sadistic

   A. Maladaptive Behavior: Difficulty in adaptively utilizing urethral sadistic patterns. This charaterizes someone who cannot start and stop quickly. He may literally be "all over the place" as far as time is concerned and has trouble knowing when he should become operational.

   Dance-Movement Therapy Techniques:

   1. Movement activities involving the rhythmic control of sharp reversals from free to bound flow which start and stop suddenly both in postural and gestural patterns. Such as activities involving quick starts and stops of a dashing nature. (All categories)
   2. Games involving running then freezing, as well as those which require knowing the right time for moving quickly. (All categories)

   B. Maladaptive Behavior: The opposite behavior can result from identification with a siginficant figure being who is fixated at this phase, or from premature bladder control. A tense pelvic area and/or constant cystitis may result. In this case the individual runs everywhere, always "doing" officiously and precisely and never allowing himself to "be."

   Dance-Movement Therapy Techniques:

   Free associational movement which first explores the somatatized conflict regarding libidinal pleasure; such as, reliving childhood dramas or the personification of and dialogue with the somatic structure. Followed by when ready movement activities which encourage urethral libidinal and inner genital libidinal rhythms. Being able to let go and allow for the experience of urethral and genital pelvic pleasurable sensations.

Related elements: Sagittal shape and time efforts, locomotor activities, semi-autonomous relationship with therapist, parallel or task group.

7. Inner Genital Libidinal

Maladaptive Behavior: Difficulty in the awareness and allowance for the experience of inner genital sensations. For example, a person may have difficulty integrating that which is unseen or may have difficulty being empirically validated into his life. In Jungian terms, he has not sufficiently integrated is anima, or feminine, side (Whitmont).

Dance-Movement Therapy Techniques:

1. Movement activities involving the rhythmic control of undulant flat wavy transitions between free and bound flow both in postural and gestural patterns. For example, movement activities of a floating nature (light, indirect, slow) or a dreamy state (lightness and free flow). (All categories)
2. Utilization of imagery or objects which would stimulate the quality such as the use of a flowing cape or sheet with slow waltz-like balletic music. (See Figure III.9.) (All categories)

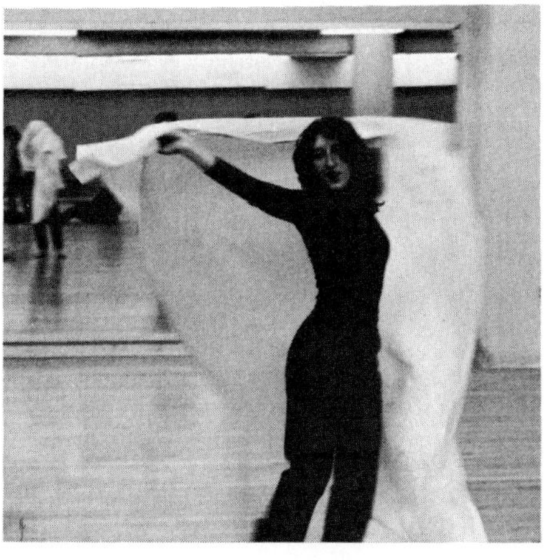

**Figure III.9.**

3. Imageful improvisations which stress themes of the organic feminine related timing in nature and within human individuation. (All categories)

   Related elements: Use of lightness, indirectness, and slowness in effort and related shape. Chumship relationship with the therapist, puberty ritual process.

8. Inner-Genital Sadistic

   Maladaptive Behavior: Difficulty in the adaptive use of feminine sadistic rhythms. For example, a woman who has difficulty facilitating delivery due to inappropriate use of movement during labor.

   Dance-Movement Therapy Techniques:

   1. Movement activities involving the rhythmic control of large undulant transitions between free and bound flow in posture and gesture. For example, movements of an expulsive nature (female).
   2. Movement activities which involve the birthing or rebirthing of aspects of a person's psychology which are ready to be integrated (Bernstein, 1980). (All categories)

      Related elements: Task group, chumship relationship with therapist, puberty and marriage ritual process.

9. Phallic Libidinal (outer genital libidinal)

   A. Maladaptive Behavior: Difficulty in the adaptive usage of phallic libidinal rhythms. This might be charcterized by a male who has not yet resolved the oedipal crisis, i.e., who has not yet formed a proper identification with a male figure or who has a highly smothering and/or seductive mother.

   Dance-Movement Therapy Techniques:

   1. Movement activities involving the rhythmic control of rounded flow adjustments with steep increases and decreases in tension. Such as movements involving penetration through an imaginary atmosphere. (All categories)
   2. Movement activities of an exhibiting and/or controlling nature. Such as have each person in the group move to the center of a circle and dance alone for a period of time (e.g., "telling us something he wants to say with his body") while the others watch. (All categories)

   B. Maladaptive Behavior: Lack of integration of the animus, or masculine, in the woman. For example, a woman who lives primarily from her unconscious and is unable to penetrate her "spaciness" with focus.

Dance-Movement Therapy Techniques:

Movement improvisations which explore various masculine animus symbols as guides for the penetration and shedding light into the unconscious. (Neurotic and other disorders)

Related elements: Chumship relationship with therapist, task group, puberty ritual process.

10. Phallic Sadistic (outer genital sadistic

Maladaptive Behavior: Difficulty in the adaptive use of phallic sadistic patterns. Such as a person who is unable to express his anger on other than a primitive level; e.g., instead of punching he bites and spits.

Dance-Movement Therapy Techniques:

1. Movements involving the rhythmic control of high intensity sharp flow reversal with steep increases and decreases in tension in both posture and gesture. For example, movements involving jumping, leaping, and driving. (All categories)
2. Use of sports activities entailing kicks, hits, bouncing balls, throwing punches, or any activity which utilizes ballistic patterns. (All categories)

Related elements: Chumship relationship with therapist, task group; Drive-object: investment of aggressive drive in external objects; use of strong, quick, direct efforts and related shape; puberty ritual process.

11. Genital Rhythm

Maladaptive Behavior: Difficulty in adaptive use of adult rhythms. This is an adult who for whatever reason has not yet evolved into a genital level of functioning. Mature sexual behavior will be difficult for him.

Dance-Movement Therapy Techniques:

1. Movement activities involving the combination of phallic and feminine inner genital rhythms producing medium intensity reversals. Such as those patterns found in everyday adult, interactional behavior. (All categories except children)
2. Movement patterns involving the central pelvic initiation of this pattern with a postural merger. For example, dancing to Afro-Carribean and rock music. (All categories except children)

3. Movement improvisations involving the personification of the masculine and feminine polarities.
   a. have individual allow for a masculine figure to emerge.
   b. have him embody the figure; let it move him and say what it needs to say.
   c. do the same with a female figure
   d. Have them interact by assuming each role.
   e. have person then explore moving in a continum from one to the other, eventually finding a middle which incorporates the two in an integrated manner. (Neurotic and other disorders where ego is present)

   Related elements: Autonomous relationship with therapist, cooperative ego-centric group, all effort-shape combinations, puberty and marriage ritual process.

## DYADIC INTERACTION LEVELS OF ORGANIZATION

Probably the most important element of the therapeutic process is the relationship established between the therapist and his patient. The success of the organization of many of the adaptive patterns is contingent upon the transference relationship. If a rapport of trust, understanding, empathy, and respect has not been constructed, it will adversely effect the total movement activity. Therefore, it is imperative that the dance therapist comprehend not only the level and needs of the individual but those of himself as well. The therapist's own needs of dependency, competition, and aggression must be satisfied outside the therapeutic relationship. Countertransference[45] must be brought to conscious awareness and utilized only if it serves the therapeutic process.

### Initial Factors in the Primary Dyadic Relationship

A neonate's normal movement repertoire takes its origin and impetus from the rhythm of his breathing. It is characterized by an alternation of growing in free flow and shrinking in bound flow. Most mothers understand this pattern intuitively and react appropriately to it. However, there are some who interpret the shrinking sequence as rejection. Due to their own feelings of inadequacy, some mothers respond by rejecting their own infants. It is very easy to perceive the spiraling effect this may have on the primary object relationship. The mother, through her movements, deprives her child of experiencing the pleasure of his body in close physical contact with his parent.

45. Countertransference: "Behavior toward the other as if the self was the original object which affect was displaced," English, from Mosey, *op. cit.*

On the other hand, if the mother is over-possessive and smothering, the movement patterns of her infant may also be adversely affected, resulting in development of maladaptive behavior in later life. This mother may respond to the shrinking movement of the neonate by continually bulging her body. If, for example, the infant shrinks momentarily from the breast in order to swallow a large amount of milk and the mother responds by bulging her breast and pushing the nipple back into his mouth, the child will choke (Kestenberg). This domineering mother denies the baby his right to sense the power and pleasure of being a separate entity. She sees the infant as an object for her own personal narcissistic pleasure. The mother needs to provide "good enough mothering" within a "facilitating environment for the maturational process" (Winnicott, 1965).

Her role is that of mediating the infant's movement through an attunement process not unlike Chace's technique of empathetic movement reflection. In this way the symbiotic relationship is encouraged. The experience of this narcissistic union is experienced both on a bodily need level and a psychic level, as it is the primary figure who not only nourishes the neonate but serves to transmit through her own psychology the child's experience of positive self existence. Winnicott (1965) stresses holding (which serves integration) and handling (which serves personalization). These body movement interactions he states, "facilitate the child's innate tendency to inhabit the body, enjoy body functions, and to accept the limitation that the skin provides a limiting membrane, separating me from not me" p. 69. In this way the separation-individuation process can occur paving the way for object constancy with the capacity for self and object and an internalized positive superego (Mahler).

### Dyadic Interaction Levels of Organization[46]

1. Egocentric—Symbiotic Object Relationship

   This is the phase of primary narcissism which follows the normal autism of the first month. It relates to the ability to perceive the mother figure when the mother figure is in the process of gratifying the needs of the self. The infant and mother exist in an omnipotent state of "dual unity" (Mahler). It is fixation at this level which results in the development of Kohut's (1971) mirror transference. (This then, is the anaclytic relationship.)

2. Object-dependent—Practicing Subphase of Separation-Individuation Process

   The individual is able to differentiate himelf from the primary object. The child commences crawling and walking but needs to check back to mother, "customs inspection" (Mahler, 1968).

46. Concepts abstracted from Mosey, Mahler, Winnicott, and Kohut.

3. Object-ambivalent—Rapprochement Subphase of Separation-Individuation Process

   The ability to trust and be dependent upon an authority figure. The individual is ambivalent about his dependency and his strivings toward independence. There is a wish for primary object to share every experience with positive regard.

4. Semi-autonomous

   The ability to explore and interact in the environment in a relatively autonomous manner though remaining primarily dependent on the parental figure for satisfaction of socio-emotional needs. The individual is required to interact with others in a protective environment while the dyadic partner continues to fulfill many of the individual's needs.[47] The individual tests the authority figure and gradually attains a sense of his own autonomy.

5. Chumship—Object Constancy

   The ability to enter into a group relationship in which the other is experienced as important to the self and the needs of the other are felt as equal to the needs of the self. The dyadic partner encourages intimate interaction between dyads or triads of individuals but is not immediately involved in the interaction. Here the individual seeks to incorporate rules and structure from the primary object, which, together with positive regard is internalized to form a realistic ego ideal.

6. Autonomous

   The ability to enter into a mutually need-satisfying relationship characterized by a firm commitment to the other which is maintained regardless of normal demands for sacrifice on the part of the self. The individual interacts in an unprotective environment and receives minimal need gratification from former dyadic partner.

## Related Maladaptive Behavior with Suggested Methods and Techniques for Dance-Movement Therapy

1. Egocentric—Symbiotic Object Relationship

   Maladaptive Behavior: Difficulty in adaptively allowing the body to merge with the dyadic figure when that person is appropriately

47. During the oedipal phase, roughly during 4–5 years of age, the triadic relationship of mother, father, and child comes into dominance. The child needs acknowledgement, recognition, and acceptance from both parents regarding his burgeoning sexuality. The child often focuses this need on the parent of the opposite sex initially. This is followed by a resolution phase in which he identifies with the same-sex parent.

satisfying the individual's basic needs. For example, this may occur if the person is unable to form a trust relationship with anyone. Autistic children characteristically are unable to relate to any human and often treat people as inanimate objects.

Dance-Movement Therapy Techniques:

1. Movement activities which involve the therapist's attuning to and merging with the rhythms and flow of the individual. This entails an adjustment on the part of the therapist to the flow and rhythmic fluctuations of the individual in a manner which will allow them to develop.

   The therapist empathetically reflects the movements of the client. This says to the person that she is not placing any demands on him and wants only to be with him where he is. Gradually a psychotic or autistic child can begin to differentiate from the therapist and view her as the source of comfort. It is only when this primary transference has been achieved that the child can re-enact maladaptive experiences. At this point the therapist can provide the needed buffering of aggressive impulses. With narcissistic personality disorders this mirroring encourages the establishment of the mirror transference in which the client assumes the therapist is "just like him" and requires of the movement therapist that she simply echo with reflective confirmation and approval the omnipotent and exhibitionistic needs of the client. Through this gradual process the grandiose self view will be contained in the movement fantasies and eventually verbally processed into reasonable ambition and action (Kohut).

2. Oral incorporative movements.[48] For example, the therapist holds the individual in a position similar to that utilized for the feeding of an infant. The therapist may then begin gradually to adapt the individual's tension flow rhythms to those of the normal sucking sequence. The therapist may also take the arms of the individual and move them in a gentle pumping fashion duplicating the neonatal associative global response to sucking. (All categories)

3. Movement activities involving the use of sounds. Although techniques may be done totally without the use of verbalization, a soothing humming or phonetic response which duplicates the rhythm being developed may also aid in reinforcing the appropriate organization of this level. (All categories)

48. See Flow Rhythms Levels of Organization; section on Oral Rhythms.

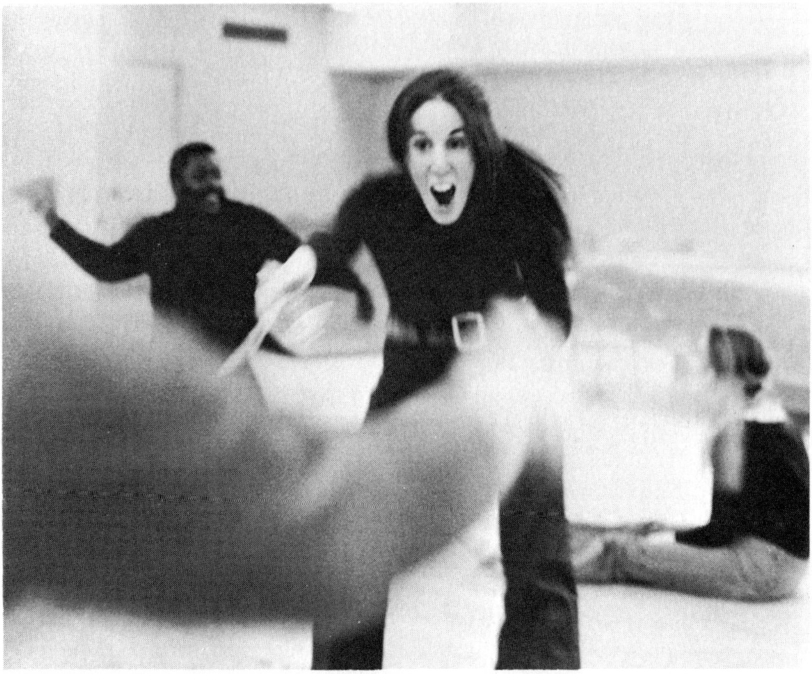

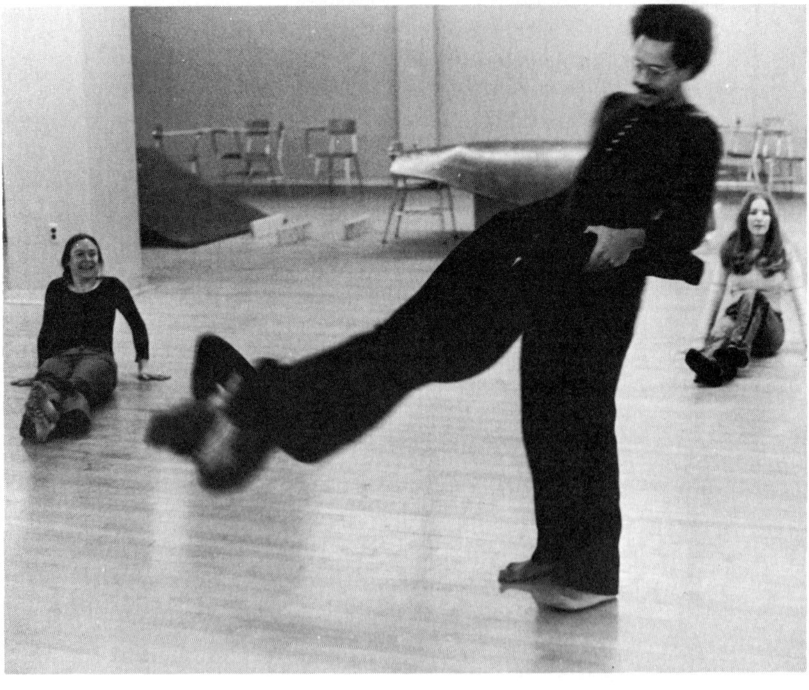

Related elements: One-to-one group, use of flow of breath, enactive level of cognition, use of tension flow and symmetrical shape flow, and investment of positive affect,[49] oral libidinal, birth ritual process.

2. Object-dependent—Practicing Subphase

A. Maladaptive Behavior: Difficulty in adaptively perceiving a differentiation between the self and the need-gratifying object; such as, the child suffering from symbiotic psychosis, who is continually merging with the therapist, falling almost limply into her arms, not sensing where the therapist ends and he begins. He may be unable to initiate a movement pattern without the physical aid of the dyadic partner, and real or imagined separation may overwhelm the ego resulting in annihilation panic (Mahler).

Dance-Movement Therapy Techniques:

Movement activities which assist the individual in perceiving the differentiation of self and therapist, and the establishment of body-image integrity and a sense of entity. For example, the therapist makes use of various forms of stimulation, such as touching (tactile), use of mirror (visual), temperature (icing), etc. (All categories, except neurotic)

B. Maladaptive Behavior: Difficulty in adaptively cessating movement patterns which are representational of those produced in the anaclytic mother-child dyad; e.g., a predominance of rocking and sucking patterns.

Dance-Movement Therapy Techniques:

Use of patterns of an oral aggressive nature.[50] Patterns such as tapping various parts of the body, or tapping the floor or therapist. Seizing and letting go of objects and imagery which makes use of blowing out of air; e.g., being the wind or a balloon, and provision of chewable food. (Children, psychotics)

Related elements: Body Image: differentiation of the body from the environment, one-to-one group, enactive level of cognition, oral aggressive rhythms, weaning ritual process.

3. Object-ambivalent—Rapprochement Subphase

Maladaptive Behavior: Inappropriate negative response to authority figures. For example, an individual who is always refusing to do

49. See Body Image Levels of Organization; Primary Level.

50. See Flow Rhythms Levels of Organization: Oral Aggressive section.

what a boss suggests at work; someone who is continually being fired because of arguments with his superior due to grandiose fantasies. This individual is unable to see authorities as both good and bad. He often has strong exhibitionistic needs to be seen and approved of as well.

Dance-Movement Therapy Techniques:

1. Movement situations which allow the client an opportunity to express negative feelings toward an authority in an imaginary movement drama which allows the client to be the victor. For example, the client may wish to recall a conflict situation between the father and himself; with a foam pillow acting as the father, the individual could slash and kick it, releasing his anger and gaining insight into his distortion of authority relationships. (Adults, neurotics)
2. Movement activities which facilitate the particular pattern for this level of organization. For example, movement activities inoving the decrease of repetition of rhythms by anticipating patterns of lower frequency and promoting a delay in their repetition.[51] (All categories)
3. Movement activities which encourage exhibitionistic narcissistic expression in contained "acting in" therapy experiences with the therapist providing needed positive regard.

   Related elements: One-to-one, parallel group, enactive or iconic levels of cognition, flow rhythms: anal sadistic.

4. Semi-autonomous

   A. Maladaptive Behavior: Difficulty in adaptively moving into a group situation; someone who, for example, shies away from any kind of group experience.

   Dance-Movement Therapy Techniques:

   Dance activities which involve the person in a small parallel group. This group would remain leader-directed. At times the therapist would respond on a one-to-one level with each of the members, similar to a class situation. (All categories)

   Related elements:

   Use of:

   Spatial pre-efforts and horizontal directional shape;

51. This decrease in the repetition of rhythms is needed for the promotion of purposeful actions (Kestenberg). See Flow Rhythms: Anal Sadistic Phase for more specific examples.

Gravitational pre-efforts and vertical directional shape;

Temporal pre-efforts and sagittal directional shape.

Enactive or iconic level of cognition.

5. Chumship—Object Constancy

Maladaptive Behavior: Difficulty in adaptively interacting with group members, lack of integration of structure and rules of group, incomplete internalization of primary object resulting in lack of realistic ego ideal.

Dance-Movement Therapy Techniques:

1. Same-sex movement groups which encourage the reinforcement of structure and themes defined and implemented by the group. (All categories)
2. Movement activities involving interaction between dyads or small subgroups of individuals which are not immediately involved with the therapist. Such as, suggest for them to explore in two's the use of a particular effort; then after a while have two dyads join together, etc., etc. (All categories)

   Related elements: spatial efforts and horizontal shaping; weight efforts and vertical shaping; temporal efforts and sagittal shaping; iconic level of cognition, task group.

6. Autonomous

Maladaptive Behavior: Difficulty in adaptively tolerating the dependency of another on the self. For example, the inability to adjust the individual's own movement patterns to those of another in a nurturing, need-satisfying relationship.

Dance-Movement Therapy Techniques:

Movement activities involving the individual in a need-satisfying role with another or other individuals—usually members of an established group.

For example, suggest to the group to form dyads, e.g., "Pair off with whoever's eyes you meet." Then involve them in a reciprocal pleasure-giving activity such as back massaging or light slapping-tapping of the partner.[52] (All categories where appropriate)

Related elements: Egocentric cooperative group, iconic and abstract level of cognition. Use of all possible effort-shape combinations.

52. Be very certain that the activity suggested is pleasure-receiving for both members.

## PRIMARY GROUP LEVELS OF ORGANIZATION

Certainly, one of the most basic adaptive behaviors needed in our society is the ability to function adequately in a variety of primary groups. The presence of an aggregate of individuals scheduled for Movement Therapy affords the therapist the opportunity to observe, evaluate, and encourage the component-related material to obtain these levels of organization. However, most groups led by dance therapists seem to remain on a basic one-to-one or parallel level of functioning.

There are often several valid reasons for group Movement Therapy being maintained at this most basic level. For example, the individuals may not be capable of functioning on a higher, more organized level; the group may not be a stable unit—members may be constantly absent or the turnover too great; the members may lack investment and involvement; the purpose, goals, or contract of the group may not be clear to its participants, producing a sense of ambiguity.

There are numerous other factors as well. However, all of the above as well as many of those not mentioned may be remedied and rendered invalid if the therapist attends to and facilitates group development reflected in gestalted group themes from movement and verbal process.

### Group Levels of Organization[53]

1. One-to-one

   As mentioned before, the one-to-one level of group functioning is the most basic. It requires the interaction of the individual with the other person (usually the therapist) either alone or in the presence of others. No demands are placed on the individual to interact in any way with the other members.

2. Parallel Group

   The parallel level requires that the individual now be able to attend to his own needs in the presence of others.

3. Task Group

   This level requires that the individual now incorporate the ability to participate in short-term tasks with others with no demands being made on him to continue the relationship outside of the designated task period. Although the leader continues to meet the emotional needs of each member, he is now responsible for encouraging interaction among the individual members.

53. Concepts abstracted from Mosey.

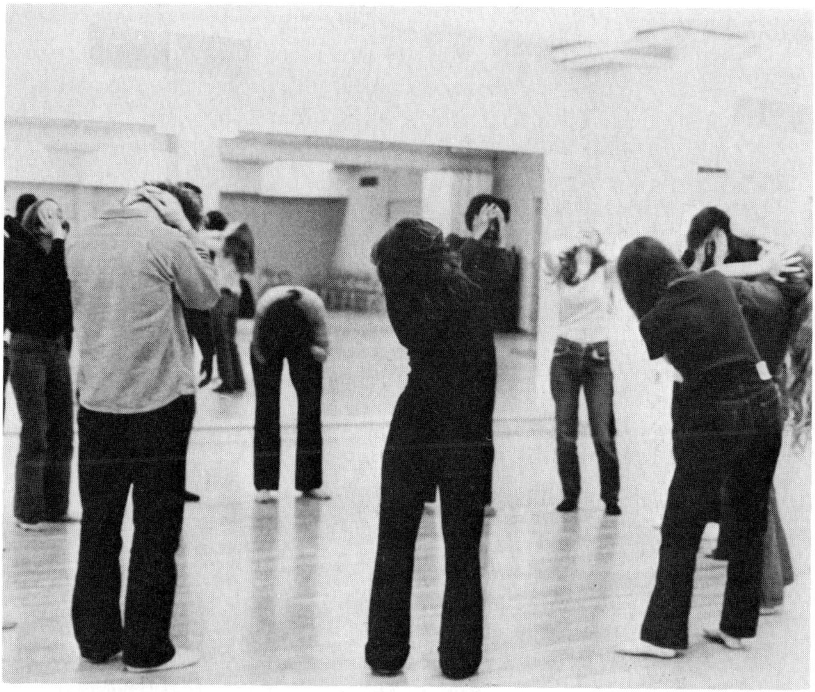

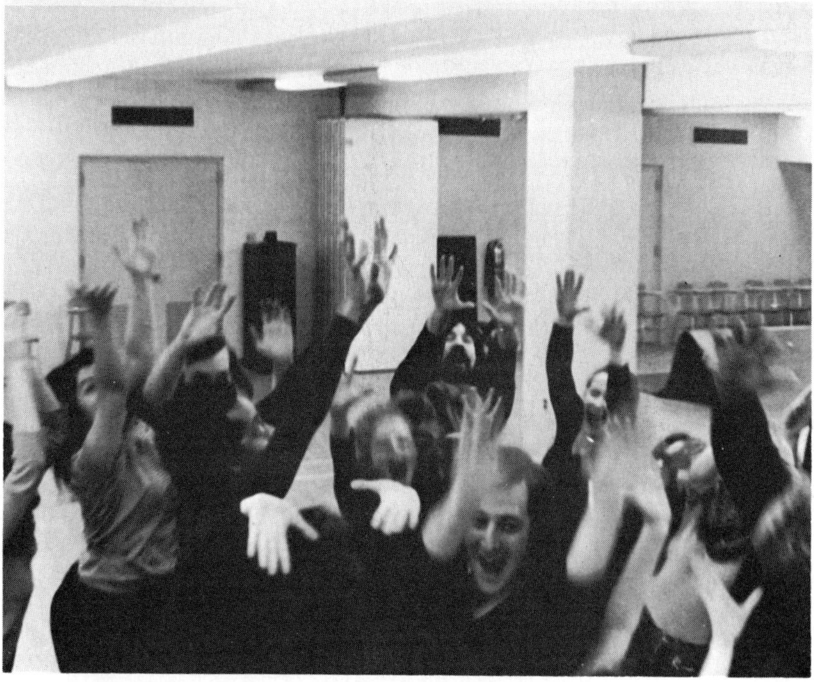

4. Egocentric and Group Cooperative

This level involves the ability to interact in a long-term task which entails not only the awareness of self interest but also the ability to satisfy defined needs of others in the group. The group is generally encouraged to make independent decisions in creating and/or exploring improvisations; however, general suggestions can be made initially when the fear of failure may be prevalent. The therapist's role is still that of support and general satisfaction of the socio-emotional needs of the members; however, with the advent of the gratification of an individual's needs by others in the group, he may evolve himself into the role of a catalyst or advisor.

## Related Maladaptive Behavior with Suggested Methods and Techniques for Dance-Movement Therapy

1. One-to-one Group

   Maladaptive Behavior: Inability to adaptively engage in Dance-Movement Therapy in the presence of others.

   Dance-Movement Therapy Techniques:

   1. Allow the individual to observe the dance therapy session. If he is unwilling to move, suggest to him that he select a record or duplicate some of the beats or patterns the group is doing while he is sitting. Let him know that even though he isn't up dancing with the rest, he is still very much a part of the group. Acknowledge his presence during the session as well as at the end. (All categories)
   2. Movement activities involving the manipulation of the individual by the therapist to promote body awareness and body image organization. For example, the therapist may stimulate the individual kinesthetically by moving his extremities through various shapes. (All categories, particularly the organically impaired)

      Related elements: Object dependent or supportive relationship with therapist, enactive or iconic level of cognition.

2. Parallel Group

   Maladaptive Behavior: Difficulty in adaptively sharing the movement session with others; a person, for example, who cannot attend to his own needs in the presence of others and will vie for the therapist's attention.

Dance-Movement Therapy Techniques:

1. Movement activities involving the meeting of the socio-emotional needs of each member. The therapist "picks up" the movement patterns of each individual and adapts them. For example, if the therapist observes a patient's movements becoming more aggressive, he may develop the sequence into a more strong, direct, quick pattern. (All categories)
2. Movement activities which involve each member attending to his own needs in the presence of others. This can be at an extremely basic level; such as, a suggestion for everyone to walk about the room at his own pace and in his own way or to give himself a message.

   Related elements: Semi-autonomous or supportive relationship with therapist; enactive or iconic level of cognition.

3. Task Group

   Maladaptive Behavior: Difficulty in adaptively involving himself in short-term tasks. This could characterize an individual who continuously moves into the center of the circle during a therapy session dancing in an exhibitionistic manner, or one who is always in competition with others for the leadership role.

   Dance-Movement Therapy Techniques:

   1. Dance sessions which afford the individual(s) an opportunity to be the leader such as when the leadership is passed around the group. (when one member is finished he passes it to a person near him and all must follow the next member's movements.) (All categories)
   2. Movement activities involving short-term tasks. For example, if the group is large divide it into subgroups and suggest a thematically related improvisation game such as charades. (All categories)

      Related elements: Supportive relationship with therapist; i.e., semi-autonomous, encouragement of chumship, enactive and/ or iconic, levels of cognition.

4. Egocentric and Group Cooperative

   Maladaptive Behavior: Difficulty in adaptively taking on a variety of membership roles. This could characterize someone who can follow well but has difficulty assuming a leadership capacity.

Dance-Movement Therapy Techniques:

1. Movement activities involving the ability of the individual to take on various roles and/or accommodate to the needs of other members. For example, each member may be given an opportunity to stage some situation that has occurred in his life that is unfinished emotionally for him; the other members of the group are used as substitutes for the actual individuals or objects involved. The individual is then allowed to propose an alternate ending to the usually emotionally charged encounter. The other members chosen to participate must be ready to act as negative or ideal figures depending on the needs of the enactor. For example, he may wish him to cower from an imaginary inflicted punch or to respond with a friendly embrace. Through this often symbolic process of resolution, the individuals will learn that they are capable of satisfying their own needs and the needs of others (Pesso). (Adults neurotics) (See Figure III.10.)
2. Use of themes that have developed from the group movement in movement dramas. (All categories)
3. Enactments of an individual's dream. Here the person is not only the writer, but the producer-director as well, selecting individuals to portray the symbols. He may wish to participate in various roles, watch it, or change it in some way.
4. Group movement dramas of myths, fairy tales, or written plays which deal with basic themes and journeys of men and women. (All categories)
5. Movement activities designed for occupational search. For example, the session may be devoted to the explaining, through active body involvement of the members, the necessary movement repertoire for a desired job, as well as role playing job interviews. (Adults, neurotics, patients leaving hospital)

   The group membership should be consistent, with an ideal range of 5–8 members.

   Related elements: Autonomous dyadic relationship, iconic and/or abstract levels of cognition.

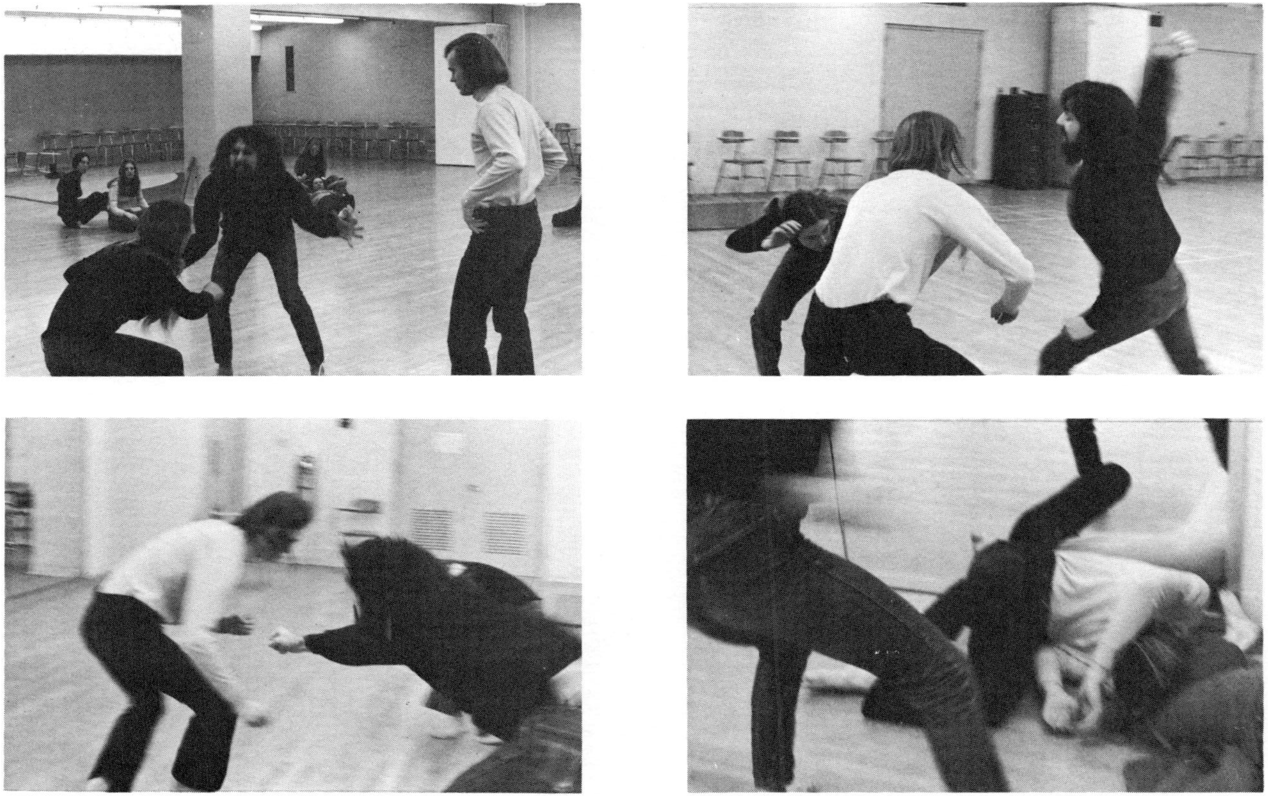

**Figure III.10.** Group cooperative: psycho-motor technique

## DRIVE-OBJECT LEVELS OF ORGANIZATION[54]

In order to satisfy primary and secondary needs,[55] an individual must be able to assemble and govern the necessary energy to acquire the appropriate need-satisfying objects. This energy, or drive, is generally considered to be in two forms: Eros related libidinal drive, which is directed toward need-fulfilling objects; and aggressive drive, which is directed toward any object that "gets in the way" of one's acquiring need-satisfaction.

Since much need gratification involves the channeling of the psychic energy through the motor apparatus, Movement Therapy is an appropriate vehicle. In movement, libidinal discharge is defined as a "type of rhythm in which 'indulging' tension flow attributes predominate." (Kestenberg, 1979, p. 144). Conversely, "fighting" tension flow attributes predominate in aggressive discharge. With each motor sequence comes a change in the inner psychic situation which serves either to bring him closer or farther away from appropriate direction of psychic energy. Increase of libidinal drive spurs growth; increase of aggressive drive spurs differentiation. It is up to the therapist to be aware of the amount of energy being expended by the client and to know whether or not the quantum allotted is appropriate for the given task. Psychic energy exists in every human being; however, because of its employment in the service of an over-used defense mechanism[56] such as repression or withdrawal, the individual may appear to be lifeless. Here all energy is expended in a somatic battle between the primitive impulse and the defending ego. Assuming that he is energyless serves only to perpetuate maladaptive behavior and further impede the free flow of energy which could be appropriately cathected and directed toward either a libidinal or aggressive object.[57]

This is one area with which dance therapists are often involved. For this reason, if for no other, it is important to have a clear picture about the necessary components needed in the acquisition of the various levels. All too often a therapist may struggle to bring about a catharsis of aggressive drive without awareness of the individual's need for libidinal investment.

54. adapted from Mosey.

55. Primary needs: nourishment, shelter, sexual satisfaction, elimination, self-esteem, reciprocal love relationship(s) (Maslow); secondary needs grow out of primary needs, such as financial security or power.

56. Defense mechanisms "are learned patterns of behavior and mental operations which help the individual to deal with conflicts between needs, drives, and cultural norms" (Mosey). They are, in other words, ego mediators between the libido (needs, drives) and the superego (rules, norms, taboos, etc.) It should also be stressed here that defense mechanisms, when utilized properly, are desired additions to a functioning ego. For example, without the mechanism of sublimation, the role of Dance Therapy would certainly be impeded.

57. A clear example of this phenomena is the person who never seems to respond in an anger-provoking situation. His body is held in a rigid bound state. It is as if he was literally using the energy in an inner battle: agonists contracted wanting to strike out and antagonists contracted keeping him from doing so due to possible fear, guilt, or a double bind situation.

## Drive Object Levels of Organization

1. Investment of Libidinal Drive in Self

   This involves the ability to place libidinal energy in the self. It is characteristic of secondary narcissism of the infant in which he perceives himself as the need gratifying object. He feels himself to be omnipotent and sees the mother figure as an extension of himself. This occurs during the symbiotic phase of object relationship.

2. Investment of Libidinal Drive in External Objects

   This involves the ability to place libidinal psychic energy in objects other than the self. The drive is first directed toward the primary object, the nurturing mother figure, and then to other objects, human as well as non-human once the capacity for self love has been established.

3. Investment of Aggressive Drive in External Objects

   This level entails the capacity to place aggressive energy in objects other than the self. The primary object is often the one to be experimented upon, especially if her attentions are directed elsewhere for a period of time. In order for this behavior to be properly integrated, the individual's use of the drive must prove to be successful to some extent. These impulses entail separating and disconnecting modes. It must also be controlled so that the individual is aware of what may be destroyed or physically affected and what should not be. Eventually splitting of the object ceases, and the capacity to invest both libidinal and aggressive drive in the same object develops.

## Related Maladaptive Behavior with Suggested Methods and Techniques for Dance Movement Therapy

1. Investment of Libidinal Drive in Self

   A. Maladaptive Behavior: Inappropriate inhibition of libidinal rhythms (usually established in infancy, such as early inhibition of autoerotic sucking).

   Dance-Movement Therapy Techniques:

   Movement activities involving the use of libidinal rhythms. Such as holding oneself and rocking to a lullaby. (All categories)

   B. Maladaptive Behavior: Non-verbal cues which suggest lack of positive self feeling; for example, unkempt clothing and hair, or poor hygenic care. These characteristics often go along with feelings of worthlessness and a flaccid limp or bound body attitude, such that there is a loss of elasticity.

Dance-Movement Therapy Techniques:

1. Activities involving tactile stimulation reinforced by positive verbalizations concerning the body. As in face-telling when the therapist touches each portion of a person's face and describes it in detail in a gentle supportive tone. E.g., "And near where your forehead ends and your eyes begin are dark brown eyebrows. They are shiny and very soft to touch. They fall in a flowing arch which follows the line of your eyes." (All categories except tactilely defensive individuals) (See Figure III.11.)
2. Movement activities involving the use of indulging pre-efforts:

   *Pre-efforts*
   flexibility
   gentleness
   hesitation
   (All categories)

   Related elements: Egocentric relationship with therapist; corresponding directional shape and shaping; flow of breath; body-image: investment of postitive affect, enactive cognition, tactile perception.

2. Investment of Libidinal Drive in External Objects

   Maladaptive Behavior: Difficulty in adaptively using indulging efforts and the corresponding shaping when with people. This then would characterize someone who might have a great deal of difficulty relating to others in a positive manner. He might relate only on an aggressive level or be unable to relate at all.

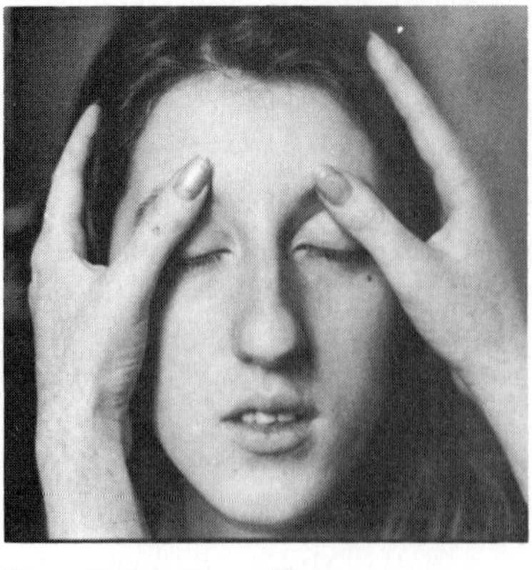

**Figure III.11.** Face telling

Dance-Movement Therapy Techniques:

Movement activities which utilize indulging efforts and corresponding shaping in various combinations in a dyadic and group experience.

| *Effort* | *Shaping* |
|---|---|
| indirect | spreading |
| light | rising |
| sustained | advancing |

Initially, the therapist may want to suggest to the group that they move toward the center of the circle using the above combinations (if age-appropriate) which might be followed by each member saying "Hello" to his fellow members when all have reached the center. (All categories)

Or the therapist may suggest that the group form dyads and have a non-verbal conversation using the above combinations. Use of a scarf or towel which both may hold is often of help, as is music with a soft flowing quality. (All categories)

Related elements: Object-dependent relationship with therapist; one-to-one or parallel group.

3. Investment of Aggressive Drive in External Objects

A. Maladaptive Behavior: A body attitude of inappropriate bound flow particularly in the jaw, shoulders, chest, and/or legs, along with insistence that the individual in question never gets angry. These people might have a great deal of fear about "letting go" with aggressive behavior. Quite often if there is no sublimated outlet for the aggressive energy, they actually feel that if they did finally "let go," they would not be able to control themselves and might destroy the environment around them.

Dance-Movement Therapy Techniques:

Movement activities involving gradual release of welled-up aggressive energy. For example, the therapist might start on a gestural level stressing the fighting efforts and corresponding shaping with which the person feels most comfortable. Gradually as the individual comes to trust his control mechanisms, the therapist can evolve him into more of a gesture-posture merging of the patterns. It is relevant to note here that if the individual does lose control and there seems to be a possibility of his hurting himself or others, the therapist may assist the person by:

1. redirecting the strong-quick-direct pattern, such as suggesting to him, "Stamp your feet," or "Hit the pillow;" or

2. evolving the individual into the utilization of more indulging qualities such as changing the attitude toward space from directness to indirectness producing a slash; or from strength to lightness producing a dab; or from quickness to sustainment producing a press; or
3. the evolving of a postural pattern into a gestural one. (All categories)

B. Maladaptive Behavior: Difficulty in adaptively moving utilizing the fighting pre-efforts and corresponding directions and the fighting efforts with corresponding shaping. This might be characteristic of a person who is described as depressed. When and if he does utilize fighting efforts, they may be always on a gestural level; or he may even turn his anger in on himself (retro-flexed rage) and take on self-mutilating behavior such as biting his nails or banging his head.

Dance-Movement Therapy Techniques:

1. Use of the fighting pre-efforts, efforts, and the corresponding shape and shaping:

| *Pre-effort* | *Directional Shape* |
|---|---|
| channeling | side across body |
| vehemence | downward |
| suddenness | backward |

| *Effort* | *Shaping* |
|---|---|
| direct | enclosing |
| strong | sinking |
| quick | retreating |

For example, gross movements such as kicking, pushing, slashing, punching, seizing, chopping, stamping, or hitting an imaginary object. (All categories)

2. Traveling movements involving getting imaginary objects out of the pathway.

For example, place pillows on the floor and have the individual kick them out of his path. He may wish to use verbalizations, such as "Get out of my way!" (All categories)

3. Circle movement activities involving release of directed aggressive energy. For example, have each member place his hands on the shoulders of the persons next to him. The circle should then gradually move from side to side with each person pushing off the shoulder of the person he is leaning toward. After momentum is built up, take the movement into the whole body. (All categories except individual). (See Figure III.12.) Or, one

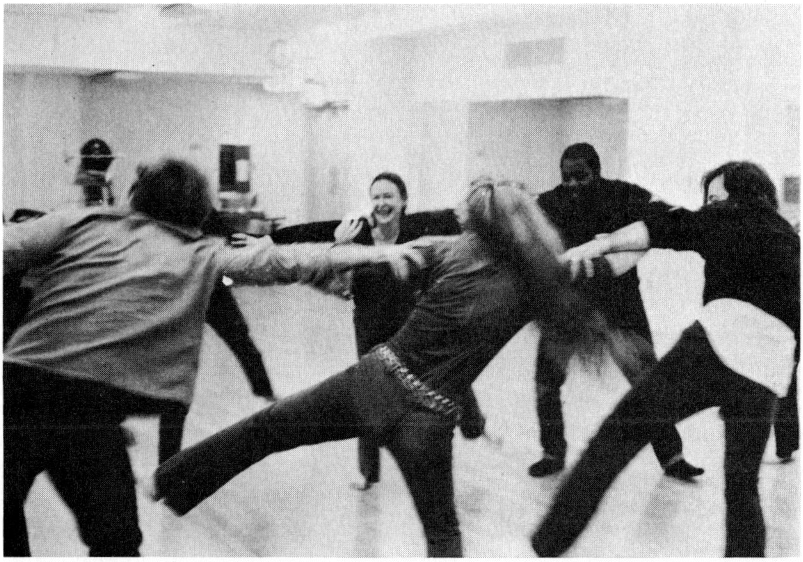

**Figure III.12.** Shoulder push-pull

individual is placed in the center of the circle; the other members close in tight. The individual is asked to get out of the circle. (Groups, adults, children, neurotic)

Related elements: Object-ambivalent, semi-autonomous, or autonomous relationship with therapist. The therapist should know when to control uncontrolled behavior and when to allow aggressive release of energy. By protecting an individual from diffuse aggressive outbursts, the person will be relieved of the guilt which would proceed from the experience (Rosen). Parallel, task, or egocentric cooperative group.

## BODY-IMAGE LEVELS OF ORGANIZATION

A healthy body image is one of the most important factors in the development of a functioning individual. It is contingent on many elements. Among them are libidinal investment in the body, awareness of the body and its functions, effective control of primary process material, and others opinion of the self including cultural norms concerning physical attractiveness.

So much of the organization of this area occurs through movement, whether it be of a purely functional or emotional basis. Paul Schilder, who conceptualized the term body-image, writes, "Motion influences the body-image and leads the person from a change in the body-image to a change in the psychic attitude."[58]

The importance of Dance-Movement Therapy is obvious. However, as with many areas of adaptive development, there exists a sequential progression of levels which must be fully organized if the person is to have an adequate body-image. Therefore, improvement in this area cannot always be assumed just because the person engages in Dance Therapy. Without sensitive awareness of the level of adaptive functioning of an individual, movement may even prove to exacerbate the existing problems. For example, on certain occasions body motion may be a destructive element in the formulation of a body-image. Movement can become a terrifying occurrence if the individual perceives his body as dissolving with every step he takes. Keeping his body silent for a period of time might be the only securing factor, particularly when he is placed in an environnent to which he is unaccustomed.[59]

Familiarity in the observation of the movement patterns through which the individual reveals his body-image is a vital and needed skill. The changes in shaping which are exhibited can tell the therapist where his focus should be in order to evolve his client to a higher, more appropriate level of functioning.

## Body Image Levels of Organization

1. Investment of Positive Affect in Body

   This level involves the capacity to perceive the body as a positive object. It entails libidinal investment in the physical properties of the self. The integration of this level is contingent upon the non-verbal communication of the primary object concerning the acceptability of the individual's body and bodily functionings, and develops from the narcissism of the symbiotic phase of object relationship.

2. Differentiation of the Body from the Environment

   This involves the capacity to perceive the difference between what is physically part of the self and what is the "other." Initially it entails the departure from the narcissistic omnipotent world of an infant with the differentiation from the primary object, the mother figure. This is followed by further disassociation from the remainder of the environment, and heralds the separation-individuation phase. Awareness of, and differentiation between, the part of the body which is internal and that which is external is also considered part of this level.

58. Paul Schilder, *The Image and Appearance of the Human Body* (Nex York: John Wiley and Sons, Inc., 1964), p. 208.

59. *Ibid.*, p. 301.

3. Recognition of Body Parts and Their Interrelationship

   This level involves the functioning knowledge of the body, its parts, and how they relate to one another. The acquisition of this ability thus entails the ability to differentiate various parts of the body in terms of their placement and function.

4. Movement of the Body Through Space

   This level entails the ability to adequately move the body through space toward a desired goal. This involves adequate motor planning as well as functioning knowledge of distance, weight, space, and time. The organization of this level is contingent upon the integration of both sides of the body freeing the individual to involve himself in activities which entail movements at and across the midline. At this stage a feeling of being the master of one's being becomes apparent.

5. Sexual Identity

   This level involves the capacity of the individual to perceive and accept his or her sexuality. This entails not only acknowledgement and libidinization of the appropriate gender but, eventually, identification with persons of the same sex as well as the capacity to choose heterosexual involvement.

   As the pubescent child progresses through adolescence, he integrates his changing body image. Growth spurts, axillary and pubic hair, development of reproductive organs—all need to be organized into his mental representation of himself.[60]

6. Aging Process

   This ongoing phase entails the recognition and acceptance of the slow, often subtle aging process which starts manifesting itself in the middle years. Awareness of the diminishing range of physical possibilities and its relationship to the need for ongoing physical conditioning are part of maintaining consciousness of this process. An appreciation for aging as a continuous growth experience toward further adult development rather than as the engendering of a negative attribute of "non-youth" is a vital component to this phenomenon.

60. Although not specified as a phase, the changes for women during pregnancy, birthing, nursing, and weaning are usually the most major body-image changes to which they must adapt. Women need to be able to tolerate and flow with the experience of nature taking control of the physical shape of their bodies. Some need to work through feelings of fear and anger regarding this process, while others deeply yearn for the psycho-physiologic hormonal reactions which allow for the more inner-genital unconscious experiences and the physical manifestation of fertility.

## Related Maladaptive Behavior with Suggested Methods and Techniques for Dance-Movement Therapy

1. Investment of Positive Affect

A. Maladaptive Behavior: Minimal or no adaptive libidinal investment in one's body. For example, there are many who perceive themselves as bad, dirty, worthless. They are continuously depressed with a slumped and/or bound body—a characteristic signal for the therapist. This means that underlying the sadness is a deep retro-flexed rage or anger turned inward. This anger might only demonstrate itself via hypochondriasis or psychosomatic complaints such as tension, ulcers, colitis, etc., but it is nonetheless very much present within the organism.[61] The anger when appropriately cathected rests with the primary object, the mother. Lack of positive interest in her child's body and in the provision of tension relieving gratification produces deep wounds to the narcissistic core.

Dance-Movement Therapy Techniques:

1. Movement activities involving adaptive tension and shape flow with gesture-posture merging, such as discussed in the Flow of Breath.
2. Movement activities designed to map out, shape, clarify, and work through dead spots or areas of somatic complaints which may be thought to hold cathectic psychic energy. For example, if the client blocks his breathing in the gut area, complains of being sick to his stomach all the time, or has continuous acid attacks, the therapist might ask the client to "look inside" his stomach and describe the feeling and what he sees. The response could be, "It's very dark, I can't see anything," or "It's like a whirlpool in there. Everything is churning around." The therapist might then ask him to pretend that this darkness could talk and to reflect about what would it say. The conversation could be helped to start by saying, e.g., "I am darkness in Fred's (client) stomach; I am here because . . ." Fred might answer, "Because I don't want Fred to know what's behind my darkness." A conversation might then develop which would lead to a movement exercise; e.g., growing into the darkness through

61. The same interpretation may be given to an individual who is always impeccably dressed, someone who spends hours getting dressed and putting on make-up, a person who wears a lot of jewelry, etc. These individuals tend to have narcissistic wounds emerging from a maladaptive ego-centric dyadic relationship (Kernberg).

to the other side, in which a greedy angry monster is revealed. (Adults, neurotics, individuals) (Gestalt)

B. Maladaptive Behavior: Difficulty in adaptively formulating interpersonal relationships. The rational for this person's difficulty is the lack of an adequate primary object relationship with the mother which showed itself in part by the mother's responding to her child as if his body were something to be touched only in a functional manner. This is the mother who may later become upset with the child's masturbatory inclinations and who usually feels negatively about her own body. Thus the client may have difficulty relating to the therapist such as those with narcissistic personality disorders.

Dance-Movement Therapy Techniques:

1. Movement activities which incorporate the therapist's touching the person's body. For example, if the client has much bound tension in his body, the therapist might have him sit in a chair or lie on a mat. She might then suggest that he relax and go limp. To test this relaxation the therapist gently picks up body parts such as the arms and passively rocks them at the shoulder joint to detect how loose and "unbound" they are. The head is also held and rolled in the socket. The therapist quietly speaks to the client telling him if the transitions are smooth or if there is a block. Reassuring the person that the therapist can hold onto the body parts without his aid is sometimes important as well. (Adults, neurotics, individuals) (See Figure III.13.)

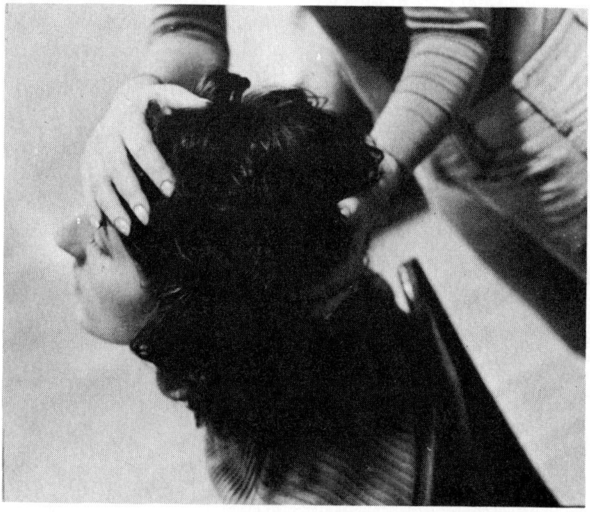

**Figure III.13.**

2. Movement activities involving gathering, grasping, and other incorporative motions. This is very workable in groups in which the acceptability of having a right to reach and take is reinforced by the other members. (All categories)
3. Dyadic movement interactions in which the individual is held. In this way the individual, through an idealizing transference (Kohut) with the movement therapist kinesthetically and emotionally, organizes an experience of being "holdable," lovable, and even a fundamental sense of existence. (Psychotics, children, and certain narcissistic personalities who have sufficient working alliances with the therapist)

Related elements: Use of oral rhythms; flow of breath; Drive object: libidinal investment in self; use of tactile stimulation, holding, and rocking; egocentric relationship with therapist; one-to-one or parallel group, weaning ritual process.

2. Differentiation of the Body from the Environment

A. Maladaptive Behavior: Body boundaries lack adaptive bound tension flow and shrinking in shape flow. This characterizes a person who is unable to differentiate his body from his surroundings. He is continually merging with the environment having regressed to or fixated at a symbiotic developmented level.

Dance-Movement Therapy Techniques:

1. Movement activities which stress the use of bound tension flow and shrinking in shape flow. Such as, gradually tensing and relaxing of various body parts in an oral aggressive rhythm or suggestions to close up tight like a ball. (All categories) (See Figure III.14.)

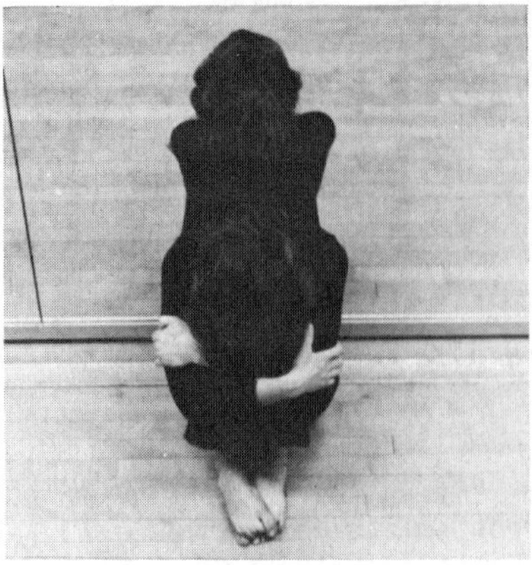

**Figure III.14.** "Like a ball."

2. Tactile and or temperature stimulation of the body using various textures such as a towel or soft brush. (All categories)
3. Activities involving the individual physically exploring that which is part of his body and that which is the "other." For example, the therapist might sit or stand with a child in front of a mirror affording him further cues. (Children, individuals, psychotics)
4. Movement activities involving verbal and physical assertion of what is the self and what is not. For example, going around a circle, one at a time, each turning to the person next to him yelling, "I am me! Who are you!" (Chace) (All categories)

B. Maladaptive Behavior: Fear that portions of the body are not attached but are floating. This characterizes an individual who has really depersonalizated; if asked to raise his arms he might refuse, and if he is able to verbalize he might say that they would drift away if he did what the therapist asked.

Dance-Movement Therapy Activities:

Techniques which involve reinforcement that the body is a totality and will not float away.

a. Have the individual view himself in a mirror (visual) or lie on the floor (tactile) and move the body part while the therapist gives proprioceptive stimulation of body part with continuous pushing of the part back into the joint; e.g., pushing arm back into shoulder joint. (All categories, appropriate for psychotics) (See Figure III.15.)
b. Pressure stimulation in which the therapist places his hands one in the front of the body and one behind. Both hands touch and leave the part simultaneously. (All categories)

C. Maladaptive Behavior: Lack of ability to distinguish between internal and external stimuli; such as with childhood psychosis in which there is no sense of individual identity and no stabilized libidinal cathexis of the body. Here the body is deanimated due to overwhelming amounts of aggressivity. Since "motion is equated with emotion, the body is projected as unhuman" and "machine-like" (Mahler, 1968, p. 36).

Dance-Movement Therapy Techniques:

Movement activities which facilitate the development of a symbiotic transference in which the movement therapist encourages first an "omnipotent dual unity" and gradually through gentile

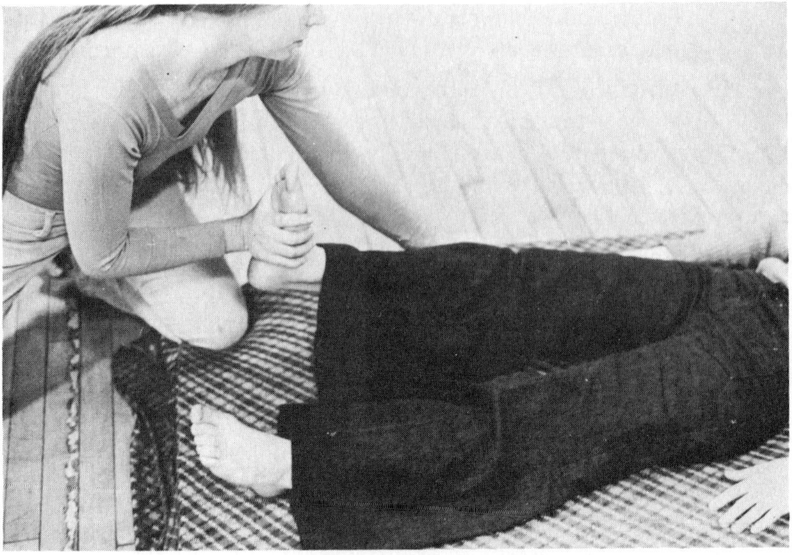

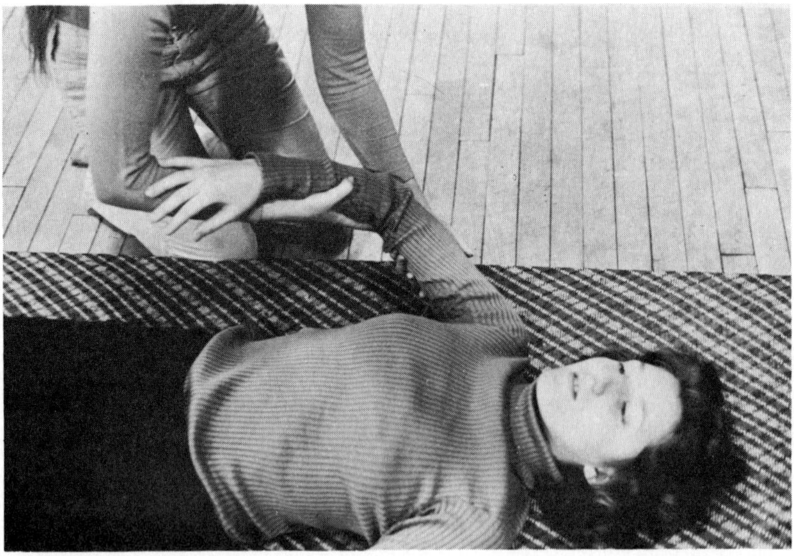

**Figure III.15.** Kinesthetic stimulation

physical stimulation, helps instill a body cohesiveness. Verbal reflection on what is internal fantasy and external reality will facilitate the organization of body boundaries. Once inner and outer is clarified, recovering the traumatic maladaptive experiences through dramatic movement fantasy enactments will assist in neutralizing the aggressivity. The contained re-experiencing within the structure of the movement therapy sessions will serve as kinesthetic prototypes for the needed developing ego apparatuses. Reinternalization of the transference object will provide further mediation through ego ideal, super ego development (Mahler, Kohut).

Related elements: Oral aggressive rhythms, regulation of tension flow and shape flow, perceptual stimulation, object-dependent relationship with therapist, one-to-one or parallel group.

3. Recognition of Body Parts and Their Interrelationship

A. Maladaptive Behavior: Cannot recognize or name body parts and/or organize their relationship.

Dance-Movement Therapy Techniques:

1. Movement activities involving the use of specific body parts, such as games similar to "Simon Says." (Children, psychotics, retarded individuals)
2. Movement activities in which the therapist inquires about the functions of body parts. For example, "Show me what a hand can do," etc. (All categories)
3. Activities involving the therapist taking a person passively through a desired pattern followed by his repeating the pattern. (All categories)
4. Dance activities involving the use of a bar, such as with leg range of motion swings. (All categories)
5. Discussion and experiential use of various body parts, nomenclature graded on complexity,

| | | | | |
|---|---|---|---|---|
| body | front | bottom | hand | waist |
| skin | back | head | shoulder | leg |
| hair | side | neck | chest | foot |
| teeth | top | arms | stomach | hip, etc., |

so that the individual may be able to touch, sight, name, experience kinesthetically, and explore the general function of them. (All categories)

6. Discussion of physical differences in a group, such as, size of feet, color of eyes, etc. (All categories)
7. Movement activities involving the use of rhythm instruments, the making of rhythm sounds by the body, and/or music; such as:
   a. Clapping, beat by tongue. (All categories)
   b. Having them establish their own rhythm; such as to their name, and see if they can duplicate each other's. (Retarded individuals, children, psychotics)
   c. Hold hands; one person sends a beat; the others pass it around the circle. (All categories)
   d. Variation exploration—quick-slow or loud-soft. (All categories)
   e. Acting out action songs. (Children, groups)

B. Maladaptive Behavior: Lack of awareness of and/or inability to recognize that which is the internal body and that which is external body. This could characterize someone who can only understand what he sees and is frightened of and/or does not understand what he cannot see.

Dance-Movement Therapy Techniques:

1. Discussion of relationship and palpation of internal and external parts of the body such as:

| | |
|---|---|
| skin | bone |
| hair | muscle |
| nails | viscera: stomach, etc. |
| teeth | fascia: fat, etc. |
| | (All categories) |

2. Activities involving the awareness of the internal body image. For example, ask the person to lie down and relax. Then suggest to him that he become aware of his breathing. Ask him then to follow the passage of air throughout his body. The therapist may mention the parts of the body in sequential fashion. The same method may be used in the digestion of an imaginary morsel of food. (All categories)

C. Maladaptive Behavior: Perceptions and distortions of the body-image. For example, body or body parts are felt to be larger or smaller, fatter or thinner, more rigid or wavy, more or less (may use self-portrait as indicator).

Dance-Movement Therapy Techniques:

1. Activities involving the creating and use of a self portrait. Such as:
   a. Have the person draw or sculpt a self-figure. Stimulus: "Draw yourself" or "make yourself with this clay." Then have him look at himself in the mirror seeing and discussing what is similar and what is dissimilar. (All categories)
   b. The therapist draws an outline of the person while he is lying on or standing next to a large full-length piece of paper (roll of brown wrapping paper is useful here). The client then draws in the rest. (All categories, especially children)
2. Autoscopy: Ask the individual to close his eyes and imagine himself standing or sitting in front of himself. Ask him to describe what he sees (Schilder). Then have him look at himself and play back for him, if possible, his description. Discuss the relationship. (Adults, individuals, neurotics)

   Related elements: Asymmetrical shape flow; pre-efforts and directional shape; perceptual stimulation; one-to-one or parallel group, object-ambivalent relationship with therapist.

4. Movement of the Body Through Space

   A. Maladaptive Behavior: Uncoordinated adaptive movement through space on a gestural and/or postural level. This characterizes someone who cannot effectively combine body parts and the relationship of the dynamics and shape of movement effectively to reach a desired goal in space or to do a task.

   Dance-Movement Therapy Techniques:

   Movement activities involving the use of effort-shape affinities and combinations. The therapist observes at which level of effort-shape organization the individual is. He also notes which qualities the individual prefers to use and develops activities around those. The therapist must always be aware of the difference between facilitating the organization of a particular attribute or quality and attempting to superimpose a novel repertoire which is not ego syntonic. (Refer to effort, shape, and posture-gesture for further specifics.) (All categories)

   B. Maladaptive Behavior: Difficulty in adaptive motor planning; for example, someone who has difficulty moving from one place to another without continuously bumping into and/or tripping over objects.

Dance-Movement Therapy Techniques:

1. Activities involving motor planning. For example, the therapist may set up a real or hypothetical obstacle course which the person must go through. He can go through forward, backward, with eyes closed, etc. (See Figure III.16.) (All categories)
2. Experience in various locomotor activities; such as hopping, walking, skipping, galloping marching, etc. (There are specific records available for these activities). (All categories)
3. Group activities which involve the following of various directions such as, "Move to the center of the circle," "Form a line," or "Move while holding your feet." These suggestions may be graded in complexity, such as, "Sit with your back against the wall and one foot on the floor." (All categories, particularly children and retarded individuals)
4. Use of related games such as musical chairs or charades. (All categories)

C. Maladaptive Behavior: Lateral dominance and/or inability to adaptively move reciprocally. This is seen when an individual is unable to cross the midline of his body. This phenomenon typically indicates organic dysfunction usually at the mid-brain level in which the primitive tonic neck reflexes were not organized and subdued by higher brain functioning (Ayres).

Dance-Movement Therapy Techniques:

Activities involving reciprocal movement as well as movement which crosses the midline of the body. For example:

a. Reciprocal swinging of arms or "bicycling" with legs when on back. (All categories)
b. Dyadic shoulder push pull: both individuals have their hands on each other's shoulder, both push with right arm then left. This same pattern can be done lying down feet to feet. (All categories)
c. Placing 2 color tile blocks or 2 color shoe prints on the floor, e.g., red for right leg blue for left. Instruct the person to follow the path stepping only on the appropriate blocks (which involve the crossing of the right over the left and the left over the right at various times). (All categories)
d. "Simon says touch your elbows." (Children)

Related elements: Effort-shape combinations, one-to-one, parallel, or task group; semi-autonomous relationship with therapist.

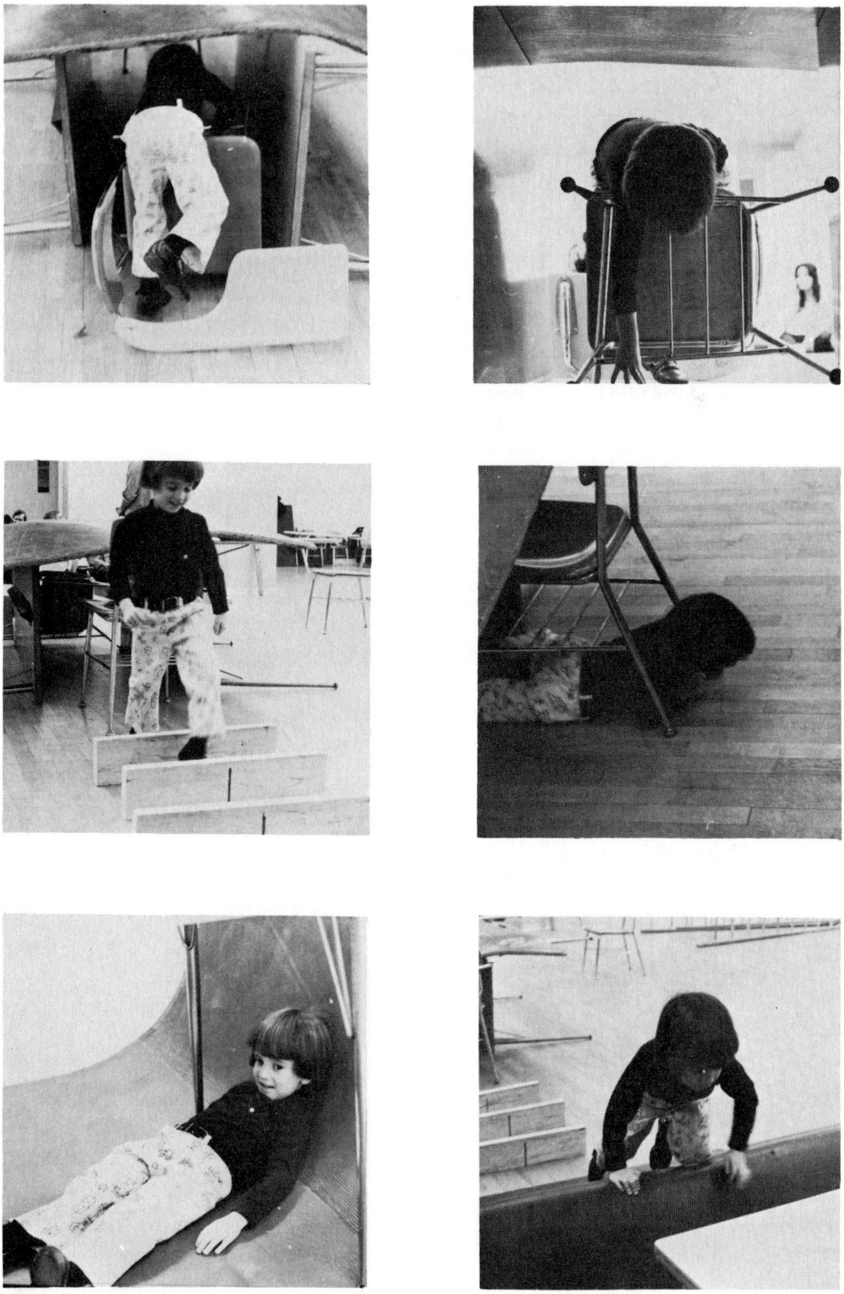

**Figure III.16.** Motor planning: obstacle course

5. Sexual Identity

A. Maladaptive Behavior: Lack of appropriate presence or difficulty with adaptive sex-specific inner-genital and outer-genital rhythms. This could characterize an individual who, for various reasons, might have either denied his or her sexuality, identified with a person of the opposite sex, or had minimal or no sexual identification with a same-sex model (asexual).

Dance-Movement Therapy Techniques:

Movement activities which emphasize the exploration of the polarities and continuum from masculine to feminine. It should be noted here that both the integration of the feminine in men (anima) and the masculine in women (animus) is a need expression of wholeness.

| *Feminine*-anima in men | *Masculine*-animus in women |
|---|---|
| inner-genital rhythms | outer-genital rhythms |
| light | strong |
| slow | quick |
| indirect | direct |
| inclusive behavior | intrusive behavior |
| enclosing, surrounding | penetrating |
| circles | leaps |
| diffuse | focus |
| unconscious | conscious |
| relating to nature | relating to societal authority |
| creative, inspirational | capacity to formulate and discriminate |
| Eros | Logos |
| cyclic | linear |
| left, yin, receptive | right, yang, active |
| creating-destroying | maintaining |
| intuition | reason |
| mystery, vision | clarity |
| time as qualitative | time as quantitative |

Use of imagery and records which are symbolic of masculine or feminine nature. (All categories)

B. Maladaptive Behavior: Maladaptive rigid posturing produced by a tense pelvic area. This person often has difficulty giving and receiving sexual gratification.

Dance-Movement Therapy Techniques:

Movement activities involving the release and movement of the pelvic area.

a. Positions which produce spontaneous movements of the pelvic area. Such as the position of hyperextension designed by Lowen. (See Figure III.17.) The thighs begin to vibrate due to muscle fatigue producing a free undulating up/down movement of the pelvis. (Adults, neurotics, individuals)

b. Dancing which involves movement of the pelvic region; e.g., Latin, rock, or African dances. (All categories)

c. Sense awareness experiences of a more subtle nature than a. or b. which seek to first explore the somatic resistences.

   (1) Draw attention to pelvic area; ask client to describe internal sensate experience.

   (2) Explore history of when the block, numbness, etc., began and discuss what was happening at that time in relation to father and mother.

   (3) Allow for any negative or positive transference to emerge in order to work through the re-enactment of past relationships and a present dyadic recapitulation of the elements needed for the resolution and organization of sexuality.

   (4) Allowance for exploration of body-felt pelvic awareness and movement. (See case of Virginia in chapter VII.)

Related elements: Semi-autonomous or autonomous relationship with therapist; parallel task, or ego-centric cooperative group, puberty ritual process.

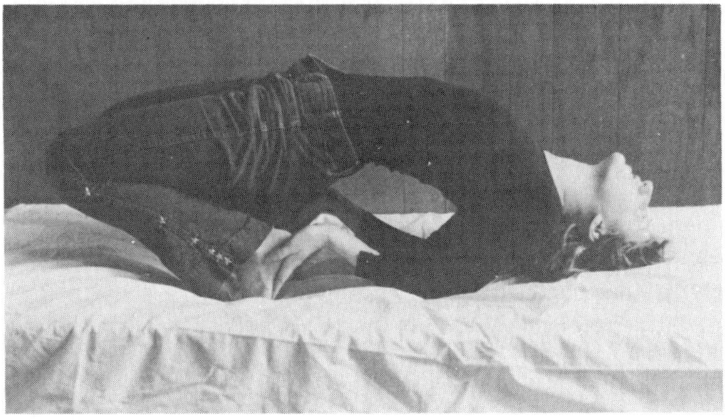

**Figure III.17.**

6. Aging Process

A. Maladaptive Behavior: Lack of acceptance of aging; engagement in activities which may be inappropriate for the person's level of physical conditioning, i.e., either underestimating or overestimating their range.

Dance-Movement Therapy Techniques:

Movement activities which encourage gradual conditioning and enlargement of physical repetoire from gestures to posture-gesture mergers.

B. Maladaptive Behavior: Denial of aging process; identification with youth via clothing, styles of relating, sexual relationships with increasingly younger individuals.

Dance-Movement Therapy Techniques:

1. Directed imagery active imagination movement improvisations which encourage the awareness and experience of the Self. (See Chapter VII.)
2. Movement improvisations employing the personification and relationship to adult archetypal animus/anima figures. Such as Sophia, prophetess, wise old woman, queen, and Great Mother (for women); and senex, guru-priest, Jupiter-Zeus, and the wise old man (for men).

Related elements: Retirement Ritual Process; Quaternary Process.

## RITES OF PASSAGE LEVELS OF ORGANIZATION

One way of looking at and working with a therapeutic developmental process is the viewing of an individual's evolution as the working through of a series of crises or milestones which correspond with key phases in the life of a human being. Society has often facilitated the progression and integration of these milestones through the use of rituals or rites of passage. Turner's *Ritual Process* elaborately states how the ritual process helps people to exist and to find their way in the complexities of organized culture. Recurrent in the work of Erikson is a fascination with how rituals introduce and aid the fledgling in becoming a member of a society at large, and then further guide the person through life and even into death.[62]

62. Penny Bernstein and Lawrence Bernstein. "A Conceptualization of Group Dance-Movement Therapy as a Ritual Process," *ADTA Monograph* Volume III. 1974.

It is quite relevant that movement is used as an avenue for rituals within therapy, since dance has traditionally been one of the most widely utilized media for rites of passage. "Rhythm facilitated the passage from one realm to the next. A dancer's step can cross the border separating life from death" (Hall, 1980, p. 110).

Role identification, replacement, and reversal, as well as basic catharsis—classic techniques in movement therapy—have all evolved from ancient ritual ceremonies. It is not surprising then that Jungian dance and psychomotor therapists have been making use of ritual for some time.[63] Whether conceptualized as an archetypal myth or a structure,[64] recapitulation of crucial periods involving symbolic rites of passage has often proven through the ages to be of therapeutic necessity.

At a time when western man has eliminated or so sapped the meaning out of what developmental ceremonies do remain, it behooves the dance movement therapist to recultivate the seeds of these processes which were sown so many years ago.

### Rites of Passage Levels of Organization

1. Birth Ritual Process

   Birth here is defined as the process through which an individual passes from a lesser to a higher, more fuller, level of life, awareness, and self-actualization.

2. Weaning Ritual Process

   The process through which an individual evolves from a state of dependence to one of autonomy, from symbiosis, through separation-individuation into experience of the self as primary need satisfyer.

3. Puberty Ritual Process

   Initiation through precept and ritual from childhood into adult life, with its corresponding sexual mores and societal demands and roles.

4. Marriage Ritual Process

   This entails a mutual commitment with another in a long-term, need-satisfying, intimate heterosexual relationship, along with the

63. Jungian Dance Therapy originated with Mary Whitehouse. See Whitehouse in Bernstein's *Eight Theoretical Approaches in Dance-Movement Therapy*. Since then others have utilized and expanded this method. See Joan Smallwood, Mary Whitehouse, Carolyn Fay, Mara Capy, and Penny Bernstein, "Five Dance Therapists Whose Life and Work Have Been Influenced by the Psychology of C. C. Jung." *American Journal of Dance Therapy*, Vol. II, No. 2, Fall/Winter 1978.

64. Structure: Pesso-Psychomotor Therapy—a motoric recapitalation of past or fantasized events in which target figures are polarized permitting expression of what was not expressed in actuality.

capacity to integrate the masculine and feminine aspects of an individual's psychology toward an intrapersonal experience of androgenous wholeness.

5. Parenthood Ritual Process

   This is a process which entails the developmental task of the wish to procreate and care for a child. This is a time-based rite of passage for the parent as well as the child in which the parents engage in the promotion and encouragement of the child's growth through the various developmental phases. Kestenberg (1974) has cited various studies which suggest that "maternal care is more gentle, soothing, and comforting; while paternal involvement is more active, exciting, and stimulating."[65] This experience is sublimated in the childless adult via the "coveted recognition of work well-done derived from the need to create, mold, and leave a perfect baby, admired by all."[66]

6. Retirement Ritual Process

   This process involves the gradual separation of an individual's active involvement within his society concomitant with a progressive feeling of ego integrity.[67]

7. Dying Ritual Process

   Death is the final rite of passage. In order for an individual to consciously and fully surrender to this experience, certain substages may need to be explored and experienced. Clearly the individual needs to be aware of the immanence of death. Denial by both the individual and the family members is often the first hurdle. Depending on the person's age and the severity of the physical problem, anger and rage may need to emerge and be expressed. The desire to "complete unfinished business," particularly with significant others, may constitute another aspect of the ritual. Finally, when acceptance of the inevitable is obtained, the individual may need to focus on his relationship to the transpersonal, the spiritual. The experience of the universal, God Consciousness, the rite of passage of the soul, as well as personal reflections and acceptance of his life, all may need to be explored before life as it is known by the person may be relinquished and death accepted as a rite of passage into another evolutionary phase of existence.

65. Judith Kestenberg, "Notes on Parenthood as a Developmental Phase," paper presented at the 1974 Amer. Psychoanalytic Assoc. Conference, p. 1

66. *Ibid.*, p. 8.

67. Ego Integrity, Erikson, *Childhood and Society*, p. 268–269.

## Related Maladaptive Behavior with Suggested Methods and Techniques for Dance-Movement Therapy

1. Birth Ritual Process

   A. Maladapture Behavior: Repressed primal fear from birth trauma characterized by fear cathected into pockets of body tension or numbered dead spots. (Blocked fear may also be represented by bulging eyes and an elevated shoulder girdle.)

   Dance-Movement Therapy Techniques:

   Movement activities involving the release of repressed fear via a recapitulation of the birth processes. A heated pool is an excellent milieu for this ritual. The designated individual should be held for several minutes in a fetal position by a mother surrogate. Eyes should be closed and the ears submerged, thereby blocking out outside stimuli. The person is moved slowly and gently through the water. Loss of consciousness will occur as sense of space, weight, and time dissipates. Other members of the group stand in two parallel lines facing each other extending from the "mother;" they act as a contracting human birth canal. Utilizing feminine sadistic rhythms throughout their bodies, they begin to push the "fetus" down the birth canal. A "doctor" stands facing the mother at the opposite end of the line and receives the individual headfirst and facilitates his grasp of reality and life by insuring that he lands upright, on his feet, grounded in reality when the birthed individual is ready to do so. (See Figure III.18.)

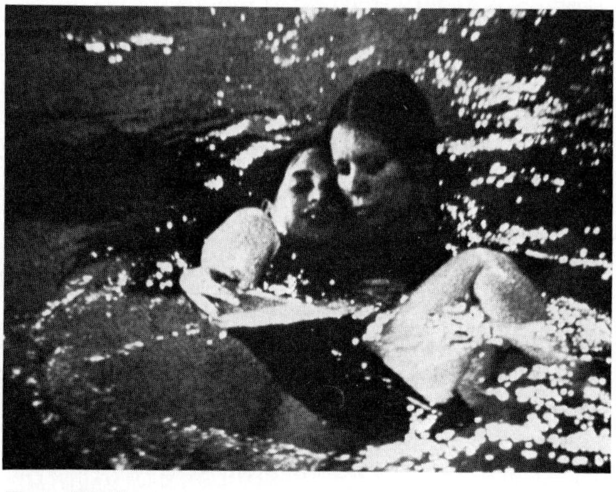

**Figure III.18.**

The individual should be allowed and encouraged to release his fear through screaming with the expelled air, which has been breathed into and released from areas tensed from repressed fear. (Normal to neurotic adults)

B. Maladaptive Behavior: Psychotic functioning which reflects a turning inward toward the retrieval and birth of some aspect of the individual's psychology through the connection with the archetypal.

Dance-Movement Therapy Techniques:

Movement therapeutic process which acknowledges, respects, and facilitates the shamanistic journey:

1. Supporting a break from the outside world;
2. Providing a buffer from being overwhelmed by the pull into the personal and collective unconscious;
3. Facilitating through movement active imagination the individual's contact with the central collective archetype and his individuation of the transpersonal perspective;
4. Guiding his return to the world and his integration and understanding of his journey in relation to his intrapsychic life and his service to humankind. (All categories particularly certain forms of essential schizophrenia, and those who through psychotropic drugs, meditation, or severe deprivation have begun the journey) (Campbell, 1972)

C. Maladaptive Behavior: Final struggles and frustration regarding the working through of a particular conflict or unintegrated aspect of his psychology. No matter what the conflict, many individuals find it difficult to evolve from maladaptive behavior to more adapture functioning even though a particular gestalt involving the integration of a prior conflict has been resolved. The process of re-aggregation,[68] or bringing the gestalt into subliminal awareness, needs a movement activity to facilitate that evolution.

Dance-Movement Therapy Techniques:

1. Movement activities involving verbal cues to the individual to facilitate a re-birth process. Such as: "You are in a small dark cave which has no room for you to stand. The way out is through

68. Re-aggregation: final stage of ritual process, see Turner, *Ritual Process*, p. 72.

a narrow tunnel. Be there, and in your own time and your own way move into the sunshine."[69] (Neurotic adults and children)

2. Movement activities involving group facilitation of the re-birth processes. Such as having group members create a womb-like environment for the individual from which he can grow from a closed to an open position. Group members may take the shape of the outside "petals" surrounding a "blossoming" individual. (All categories)

   Related elements: Breath flow, symmetrical shape flow, inner genital sadistic rhythm.

2. Weaning Ritual Process

   A. Maladaptive Behavior: Life seems to be too painful, and basic trust seems to be unavailable to the individual who was not provided with good enough mothering for the weaning process to complete itself. He cannot seem to initiate any dyadic movement experiences when involved in group dance improvisations. The person may continuously place himself in a passive role in relationship to others, merge or exhibit grandiose, narcissistic, and/or exhibitionistic behavior in sessions.

   Dance-Movement Therapy Techniques:

   Dyadic movement rites involving the nurturing and rocking of the individual with empathetic acceptance within an idealized or mirror transference. This may be graded such that more initiative in movement exploration and interaction is developed and reinforced by the therapist as the individual moves into the rapprochement phases of weaning.[70] (All categories)

   B. Maladaptive Behavior: Inability to "take a stand" in relation to authority figures, characterized by repressed hostility toward one or more parents. The individual is often fixated at an anal ambivalent phase exhibiting excessive use of the anal libidinal rhythm in pure and mixed form.

   Dance-Movement Therapy Techniques:

   1. Movement activities involving an autonomy rite of passage. In order for the individual to feel comfortable about expressing

69. Quite often the individual will evolve into this rebirth process on his own as the natural resolution and completion of a previously conflicted area. The ritual is easily detected during verbal sharing at the end of the session. See Bernstein's "A Mythologic Quest: Jungian Dance Therapy with the Psychosomatic Client." *American Journal of Dance Therapy*, Vol. 3, no. 2, Spring 1980.

70. Albert Pesso, *Experience in Action.*

repressed anger toward parental figures, each parent is split in two; some group members become bad parents and others become his good parents supporting him in his cathartic expression of anger. Support may be both physical and verbal (Pesso). The good parents may even initially help him emote by evolving him into strong, quick, direct patterns through synchronous, evolutionary movement (Chace). The negative accomodators, or "bad parents," may encourage the enactor's angry release by saying that they are model parents, or by denying every accusation (psychodrama). If they prove to be too strong adversaries, they can be instructed to cringe and whimper at even the mere suggestion of strength exhibited by the individual. The ritual may be completed by the enactor destroying the bad parents with the reinforcement and love from the good parents. This splitting is pathological however. The individual needs to be able to view his parents as both good and bad. (Adult neurotics)

2. Movement activity involving the ritual making and subsequent destruction of a life-size "mother." (Adults and children, but when used with children, the figure need not necessarily be identified.)
3. Movement-drama activities in which the individual becomes the parent or symbolic figure of power. Quite often children will become monsters or wild animals capable of devouring and thereby incorporating the powerful therapists or any other authority figures. This identification with and incorporation of the aggressor and has been utilized in rituals throughout time in hunting cultures. (Children)

   Related elements: Oral libidinal, anal sadistic flow rhythms, investment of postive affect, egocentric and object ambivalent relationship.

3. Puberty Ritual Process:

   A. Maladaptive Behavior: Role confusion with lack of a sense of identification within the transition from childhood to adulthood which may show itself behaviorally in immature child-like movements, excessive amounts of tension flow with difficulty in moving utilizing full-effort actions. Clothing or self-drawing may be asexual and/or infantile.

   Dance-Movement Therapy Techniques:

   1. Movement drama activities involving the trying on of numerous identities through the role-playing of a variety of adult figures

which may be ego ideals or heroes of the individuals. Other group members may be asked to respond in previously designated manners to the particular individual. (Adolescents)

2. Movement activities involving reenactment of myths or culturally appropriate stories of adolescents who become adults through a particular rite or deed. A group or individual may wish to create and move through their own pubescent rite of passage. With just a few verbal cues from the therapist, such as "allow your body to sculpt itself as you were as a child . . . and now as you will be as an adult. Now move from the child position-pattern to those of an adult, being aware of the evolutionary process" a ritual process may be created. Or have a group plan and carry out or improvise their own ceremonial puberty dance. (Age-appropriate population)[71]
3. Enactments of fairytales such as "Cinderella," "The Princess and the Frog," and "Snow White" which speak to the resolution of the puberty ritual process. (All categories)

B. Maladaptive Behavior: Inability to have an adequate sexual relationship due to lack of resolution of the oedipal crisis.[72] In males this may show itself in a dual hatred of and sexual attraction to women.

Dance-Movement Therapy Techniques:

1. Movement ritual process involving the working through of oedipal stirrings. Here again the accomodators may de divided into positive and negative "parents." The negative parent of the opposite sex responds seductively to the enactor-individual. In the case of a male-identified patient, the good father responds by not permitting any form of sexual interaction to occur with the bad mother. Verbalizations such as "We understand your desire to seduce your mother, but we will not allow that to happen." Father: "Only I have sexual intercourse with your mother." A positive, more age-appropriate sexual companion is often provided in this type of psychomotor structure. Resolution comes when the enactor-individual realizes that he cannot have his mother even though she may have been seductive and that a woman close to his own age is more appropriate for him. This same structure may be reversed for an electra ritual in

71. See case study of Mark in Chapter X.

72. Puberty has often been called the Second Oedipal phase due to emerging sexuality and a resurgence of interest in the parent of the opposite sex.

which the bad father attempts to seduce the daughter.[73] (Neurotics)

2. Enactments of myths and fairytales which explore and speak to this theme. (All categories)

   Related elements: Full efforts, P-G merger, phallic and feminine rhythms, sexual identity.

4. Marriage Ritual Process

   A. Maladaptive Behavior: Inability to sustain a lasting intimate heterosexual relationship which may show itself in difficulty in commitment (diminished use of the vertical plane) and closed shape flow characteristic of the puer and puella aeterni. Urethral sadistic rhythms and/or quickness and free flow may dominate the individual's repertoire. Lack of an abundance of adult genital rhythms may also be apparent.

   Dance-Movement Therapy Techniques:

   1. Movement activities involving a symbolic ritual union between two individuals. The rhythm and flow of such an activity may be evolved intuitively, being aware each moment of the goal of union and of what the person is feeling in relation to his own energy and the energy of the partner. The ritual terminates when they have sculpted their bodies in appropriate relation to the other. (All adult population) (See Figure III.19.)
   2. Since it is important to understand that dualism is an illusion, particularly when involved in a heterosexual relationship, movement rituals involving role reversals and/or calling forth his anima (for the man) and her animus (for the woman) may be highly important.[74] At first each of the dyad may wish to move alone, but eventually it would be important to interact and thereby gain a total awareness of the multiplicity of the yin/yang relationship which exists. (Normal-neurotic adults)
   3. Movement ritual which involves the use of stimuli such as African or Afro-Caribbean music which simulates the sexual encounter and relationship. This may take the form of fertility rites which have existed in many primal cultures. (Normal-neurotic adults)

73. Pesso.

74. Animus: (C. G. Jung) The archetype that is the masculine component of all women's personalities resulting from accumulated racial experiences of women with men. Anima: femine component. (Wolman)

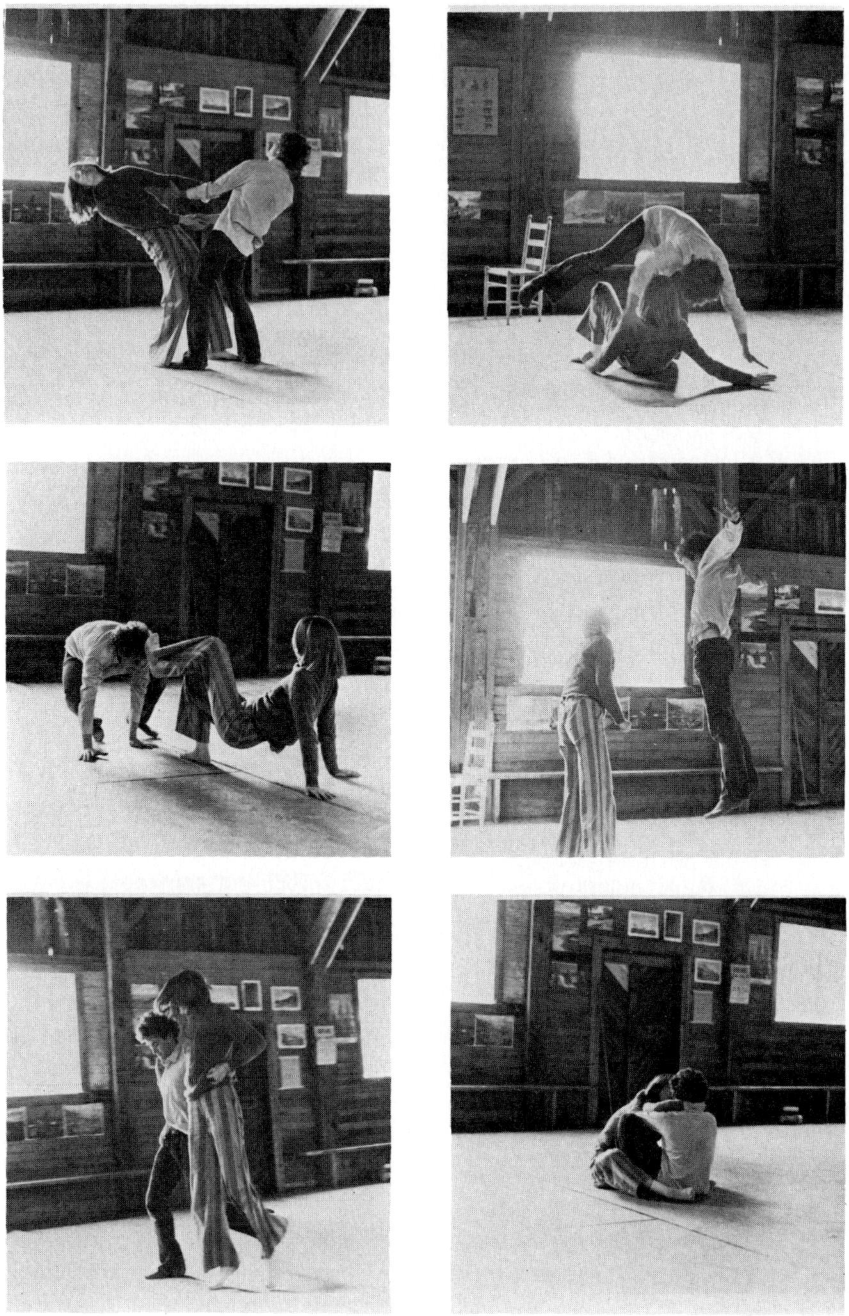

**Figure III.19.** Marriage ritual

B. Maladaptive Behavior: Lack of intrapsychic integration of the masculine and feminine within an individual. This may take the form of an animus possessed woman who relates to the world with a predominence of fighting efforts or an anima possessed man whose brooding moodiness deters him from penetrating the world.

Dance-Movement Therapy Techniques:

Movement active imagination which explores dialogues and personifications of various animi and animae archetypes; such as Demeter, Amazon, moon mother, virgin, witch, priestess for women and Zeus, Apollo, sun god, sorcerer, guru for men. (All categories)

Related Elements: Adult genital rhythms.

5. Parenthood Ritual Process

A. Maladaptive Behavior: Lack of drive toward creating, whether it be a child or a product.

Dance-Movement Therapy Techniques:

1. Movement activities which focus on and encourage the individual's utilization of the creative process. Use of improvisational dance, free associations, poetry, drawing, and other artistic expressions may stimulate psycho-physiologic processes. (All categories)
2. Active imagination thematic body-movement images which focus on the individual's fertility and potency. (All age-appropriate populations)

B. Maladaptive Behavior: Dyadic verbal and nonverbal behavior which denotes lack of organization of identification with "good enough" parental role models in their own development.

Dance-Movement Therapy Techniques:

Total movement activities which engage the individual in a dyadic transferential relationship allowing for:

a. Awareness of experiences of negative parental role model during childhood.
b. Exploration and reinactment of negative environment, associated feelings, and any negative transference.
c. Development of positive maternal or paternal transference along with facilitation of environment which encourages related developmentally based experiences.

d. Identification and integration of positive transference figure. (See Chapter VIII on role of the therapist for further delineation.) (Individuals capable of forming a working alliance)

Related elements: Genital rhythms.

6. Retirement Ritual Process

Maladaptive Behavior: Despair and depression are often characterized by a giving-in flaccidity (hopelessness, helplessness) or a tensely bound body (depression, repressed anger, and sadness) due to feelings of loss instigated through a sense of loss of oneself—one's life. Alienation and sense of separateness may manifest itself via a decreased use of shaping and a hollowed, shortened, and/or narrowed torso.

Dance-Movement Therapy Techniques:

1. Movement ritual involving the tapping into and discovery of unconscious archetypal movement patterns which stem from a collective unconscious. These patterns which have a universal-infinite quality should be encouraged and allowed to develop. Learned movement patterns which were formerly associated with previous personae and/or jobs should be discouraged. It is important that some individuals understand that the latter patterns are not always an integral part of their being, and that the possible sensations of loss of oneself due to loss of job identities may really be anthetical to what is actually the case, i.e., they may now, for the first time, really be availing themselves to the possibility of being who they are. (Normal-neurotic appropriate age)
2. Movement activities involving the dissolution of body ego boundaries and the encouragement of a sense of oneness and unity with the environment. Such as a group moving in a heated pool in a clump-like mass. Individuals may be carried by others. Total relaxation is encouraged as the group takes on the form of a human seaweed. (Normal-neurotic adults) Verbal cues which stimulate body relaxation and peak experiences, yoga, T'ai Chi Chuan, and other forms of movement meditation may also be suggested. (All age-appropriate populations with enough ego boundaries)

7. Dying Ritual Process

A. Maladaptive Behavior: Denial of dying or of anger concerning one's death; concern for others as a defense against turning inward to self-exploration.

Dance-Movement Therapy Techniques:

1. Use of imagery which allows for the individual to go into his body and locate the disease, dysfunction, or spector of death within him; personify it; and hear what it has to say to him. This process may aid in bringing to consciousness what his body already knows. (All appropriate populations)
2. Empathetic verbal reflection, acknowledgement of space and time given for the individual to express his feelings regarding his death. Depending on the form of the illness and precautions, movement may or may not be appropriate. However, verbal expression with assurance of a horizontally aligned body posture and breathing which is in service to the expression are viable techniques for this process. (Those who are dying)

B. Maladaptive Behavior: Difficulty in working though "unfinished business" in relationships with significant others.

Dance-Movement Therapy Techniques:

Facilitation of communication between the patient and the individual in question, along with encouragement of physical touch and body relatedness. (People often find it difficult to accept the death of others because it forces them to deal with their own mortality. Not wanting to touch a dying person is a manifestation of not wanting to be in contact with the utimate fate of all life forms.) If the significant other is not present, facilitate the individual's "bringing him into the room" and telling him what he needs to share. (All categories with ego)

C. Maladaptive Behavior: Difficulty in fully relating to the bridge to the beyond, the spiritual, the soul, and/or the universal.

Dance-Movement Therapy Techniques:

1. Use of guided imagery and directed fantasy which seeks to contact the higher self, the soul, and its relationship to that which never dies but only changes. (See Psychosynthesis literature for suggestions.) (All populations)
2. Encourage a psychic and bodily fantasy of death and what the individual envisions the rite of passage upon death will be like. (All populations)
3. Suggest that the person image a significant other in his life who has died. Have him ask the person any questions he may have and allow for the figure to be a guide.

4. Readings from the Tibetan Book of the Dead with suggestions for bodily felt imaging of the various post mortem stages may be appropriate depending on the individual's belief system.

Related elements: Quaternary Process.

## TACTILE PERCEPTUAL LEVELS OF ORGANIZATION

In order to react to and adaptively move in an environment, an individual must first be able to perceive it appropriately. If he is unable to do so, due to neuromuscular impairment and/or an environment which has not supplied an adequate amount of stimuli, the individual will be severely impeded in his attempts to learn and integrate other adaptive patterns.

Perception of tactile stimulation is one of the first avenues open to an infant. In the womb, he reacts to stimuli produced by the grosser movements of the mother which penetrate his nirvana. After birth, the neonate continues to respond to stimulation which, for the most part, is initiated by the mother or mother surrogate. Her ministerings to her child's needs serve to build a reservoir of various tactile experiences which are recorded and responded to at an emotive level. This data affords the infant some of the basic elements needed in the process of differentiating himself first from his mother and then from the rest of his environment. Without this ability, as seen particularly with autistic children and severely regressed schizophrenics, the individual cannot perceive where his being ends and the outside world begins—a situation which renders functioning, even at the most basic level, impossible. Faulty handling results in poor muscle tone, maladaptive coordination, difficulty in experiencing body functioning and depersonalization i.e. a split between the ego and the body (Winnicott, 1965).

The importance of this adaptive pattern, however, is often not matched by the degree of interest and attention therapists and educators place upon it. In a strict sense it could be argued that integration of tactile perception, or of any other form of perception for that matter, is not and should not be part of the role of the dance therapist. He should involve himself solely with the client's movement patterns and leave the integration of perceptual skills to someone else.

On the surface, this argument certainly has validity if there were other therapists who could work with the client in this area. However, unfortunately there are very few psychotherapists who work at this level. Since it is an area which cannot be overlooked or discarded as unimportant to motor development and the organization of adaptive levels, the movement therapist carefully attends to this area. It must also be noted that the dance therapist, among all other psychotherapists, is best equipped to handle and treat this most basic and vitally important area.

The importance of the use of tactile stimulation cannot be over emphasized in the work of the dance therapist. As with the dancer, the major tool of the therapist is the body. It is the primary communicative device through which the therapist and his client relate and work. Stimulation of the body serves to communicate to the respondent, and often to the stimulator as well, fundamental information which is imperative to the therapeutic process.

For example, the therapist may not only use tactile stimulation to aid the individual in the acquisition of this perceptual ability on the feeling of being "touchable," but also as a diagnostic tool. He may sense if the body is tense, rigid, or lifeless. If, for example, a cold area is detected without any apparent environmental reason, it might suggest an area charged with cathected energy. A light stroke over the torso might detect a difference in body quality which would suggest a disassociation of one portion of the body from the other such as is found with the "cutting off" of the pelvic area due to sexual psychopathology.[75]

The use of physical contact and tactile stimulation in the development of interpersonal relationships is or should be obvious to every human being, whether it be a hand shake from a friend, a nurturing stroke from a mother,

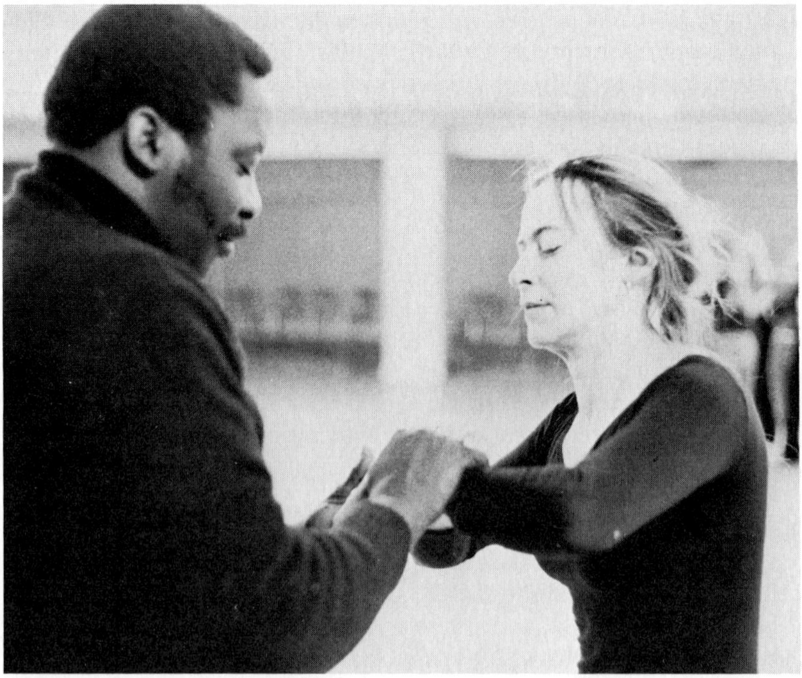

75. Alexander Lowen, "Thinking and Feeling," Lecture Reprint, 1967.

or a caress from a lover. Because of its direct primitive communicative nature, some psychotherapists have made use of it to relate to those individuals who might not otherwise respond. It is only natural that movement therapists utilize this method in establishing relationships with those individuals who are in need of this basic level of reassurance. A dance therapist who refuses to do so may reinforce a person's concept of himself as an "untouchable worthless creature" as well as decrease the chances of his integrating needed adaptive patterns particularly at the narcissistic levels of development discussed by Mahler, Kohut, Winnicott, Kernberg, et al.

### Tactile Perceptual Levels of Organization

1. Tactile Recognition

   This level entails the capacity to recognize or sense tactile stimulation. Recognition generally takes the form of a response of some kind, such as a verbal affirmation or a motor reaction.

2. Tactile Discrimination

   This level involves the ability to discriminate one tactile stimulus from another. The stimuli may differ in degree of pressure, texture, temperature, or area of the body, as well as in their emotive quality. When the latter quality is involved, the response takes the form of either approaching (with a pleasant stimulus) or withdrawing from (with a noxious stimulus). This last ability is vital to appropriate object relationship formulations and therefore cannot be overlooked.

3. Tactile Retention and Recall

   This last level involves the ability to hold in memory the tactile stimulation. This entails the capacity to remember the form and quality of the stimuli as well as the previous appropriate response to it. This level is vital for the incorporation of the primary feelings of being lovable and worthy of being touched by the significant other.

### Related Maladaptive Behavior with Suggested Methods and Techniques for Dance-Movement Therapy

1. Tactile Recognition

   A. Maladaptive Behavior: Inappropriate use of flow. For example, a body which seems to be "too flexible" often permits stimulation to pass through the outside membrane without the necessary body ego control; or a body which seems to be "too rigid," due to the individual's desire to totally withdraw from reality, attempts to "desensitize" receptor systems so as not to receive any cues which might bring the individual into closer contact with his environment.

Dance-Movement Therapy Techniques:

Dance-movement activities which make use of the qualities of tension and shape flow along with gentle tactile stimulation acts as a normalizing buffer between inner and outer and aids in development of a libidinized body perifery. (See corresponding section.)

B. Maladaptive Behavior: Difficulty or lack of adaptive response to tactile stimulation. A good example of this phenomenon is the frequent response, or rather lack of response, of the autistic child to the humans around him.

Dance-Movement Therapy Techniques:

1. Movement activity involving general temperotactile stimulation such as with a cold cloth or ice. Sensory stimulation should at least initially harmonize with the natural rhythm of the person. If a pool is available, it can be utilized in this area. Depending on the level of the client, the therapist may wish to hold him simulating in utero and work toward drawing him into free and independent movement in the water.[76] (All categories)
2. Movement activity involving the therapist's holding the individual, usually coupled with rocking. The therapist may hold the client in a nurturing, comforting manner; or, if the individual is in a hysterical or explosive state and needs to sense a stronger more securing involvement with the therapist, he may position the individual in his lap so that the client's back is to the therapist. The arms of the child are crossed and the hands held. If he is kicking, as in an uncontrolled tantrum state, the therapist may wish to wrap his legs over those of the individual. He should not be held too tightly; some degree of movement can still be allowed to take place. Gradually, the therapist can work toward drawing the high degree of motion into slower, more subtle activity. Breathing can also be duplicated by the

76. This nurturant holding of the individual is particularly important if the patient demonstrates any signs of body image diffusion. It is best never to force anyone into this milieu, as doing so could prove to have a highly damaging effect.

therapist and decreased slowly to a more normal rate.[77] (Children) (See Figure III.20.)

C. Maladaptive Behavior: Tactile defensiveness such as that which is often due to repressed rage and fear of the stimulator as well as of his reaction to the stimulus.

Dance-Movement Therapy Techniques:

1. Activities in which the individual himself does the initial stimulation, gradually followed by the therapist becoming involved. For example, vigorous but gentle slapping or tapping of body followed by rest for sensing. (All categories)
2. Movement activities which aid the individual in releasing the suppressed rage (such as those discussed previously in Drive-Object: external investment of aggressive drive).

   Related elements: Egocentric relationship; one-to-one or parallel group.

2. Tactile Discrimination

   A. Maladaptive Behavior: Difficulty with adaptive texture, temperature, and/or pressure discrimination. Such as a child who cannot tell the difference between a smooth and rough surface.

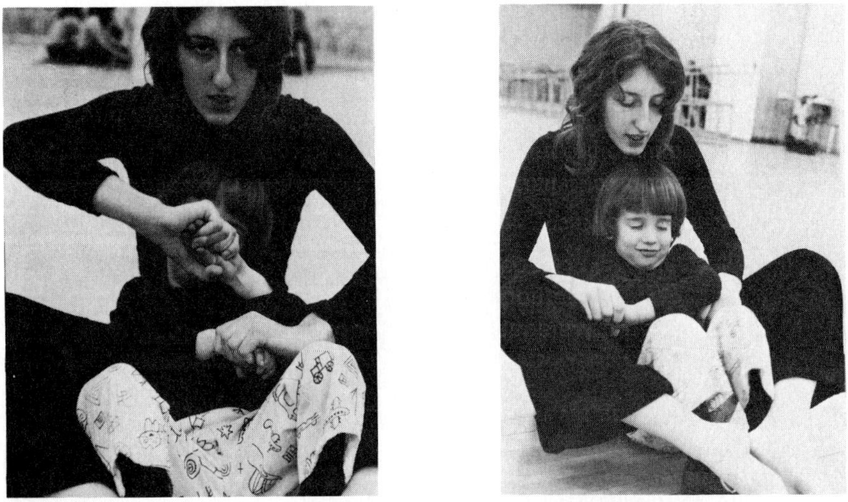

**Figure III.20.**

77. It is important not to overuse this method, particularly when the individual is working toward ego control, lest the developing ego will be damaged. A good therapist senses when it is appropriate to hold and when not to. Reinforcing dependent behavior may cripple a client and keep him in a dependent transference with the therapist.

Dance-Movement Therapy Techniques:

Activities involving the discrimination of various tactile stimuli involving degrees of pressure, texture, temperature, or area of the body; use of cloth, brushes, sandpaper, and various other textures. For example, if the therapist were to work with the child mentioned above, he might make use of various textures of floor tiles. Graded in difficulty, he might lay out several pairs of textures and have the child while blindfolded match the pairs using either hands or feet to touch the tiles. (All categories when applicable) (See Figure III.21.)

B. Maladaptive Behavior: Inability to adaptively differentiate between positive and noxious stimuli. For example, an individual who responds by growing toward a negative tactile stimulus.

Dance-Movement Therapy Techniques:

Activities involving the discrimination of pleasant from unpleasant tactile stimuli by motor response, such as those discussed in the organization of asymmetrical shape flow.

Related elements: Object dependent or object-ambivalent relationship with the therapist. One-to-one, parallel, or task group.

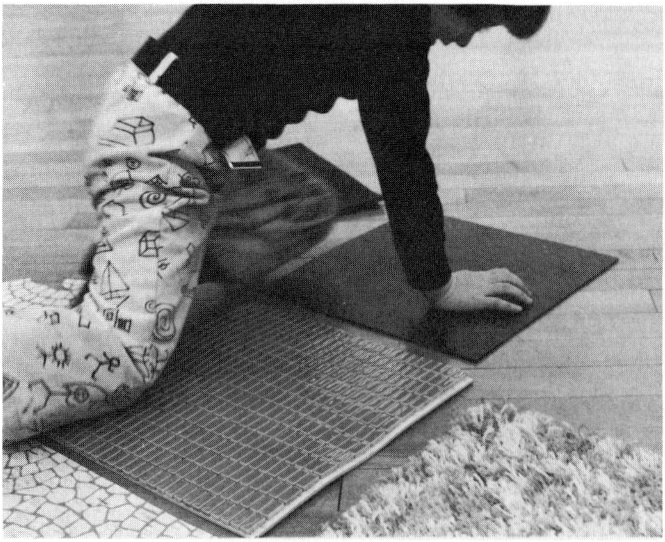

**Figure III.21.** Texture discrimination

3. Tactile Retention and Recall

Maladaptive Behavior: Difficulty or inability in adaptively remembering the form and quality of past tactile stimulation.

Dance-Movement Therapy Techniques:

Activities involving first the stimulation of a part of the body, and then, after an extendable period of time, the individual's responses as to the area, form, and quality of the stimuli. (All categories)

Related elements: Object-ambivalent or semi-autonomous relationship with therapist; one-to-one, parallel, or task group.

## KINESTHETIC PERCEPTUAL LEVELS OF ORGANIZATION

If the body is to move in a functional manner, an individual must be able to sense internally as well as externally. He must know unconsciously what position his extremities are in in order to make even the most insignificant purposeful movement. If he does not have this capacity, he must diligently watch every move, and even then his movements are uncoordinated and perhaps athetoid in nature.

Movement of this type usually suggests certain forms of brain damage. However, if an individual is severely regressed to an infantile state, or even if he has unconsciously desensitized a portion of his body, his proprioceptors and vibratory receptors may react as if there were organic impairment. Blind individuals need particular involvement with this constellation. The kinesthetic system is composed of the proprioceptive and vibratory senses; specifically, proprioception involves the mediation of position sense, sense of movement, and deep pressure sense, as well as aiding in equilibration. At least four types of receptors of this kind are located in the joints, tendons, and muscles. Their position alone justifies the attention of the movement therapist.

Vibration sense, although not as important a sense mechanism as proprioception, is still a useful detective system particularly when employed by the movement therapist.

Kinesthetic sense along with other basic forms of perception constitute the major vehicles for the development of a stabilized body-image within the symbiotic and separation-individuation phases of object relationship. Mahler (1968) writes, "Proprioceptive inner stimuli . . . in the nursing situation contributes much more importantly and immediately to the body-image than do the later maturing distance perceptive, visual and auditory images" p. 36.

### Kinesthetic Perceptual Levels of Organization

1. Kinesthetic Recognition

   This level involves the capacity to recognize or sense proprioceptive and vibratory stimulation. Recognition may take the form of a verbal affirmation or motor reaction.

2. Kinesthetic Discrimination

   This level involves the ability to discriminate and localize proprioceptive and vibratory stimulation.

3. Kinesthetic Retention and Recall

   This level involves the capacity to hold in memory the proprioceptive and/or vibratory quality of the stimuli and to duplicate it by reconstructing the movement pattern which produced it.

### Related Maladaptive Behavior with Suggested Methods and Techniques for Dance-Movement Therapy

1. Kinesthetic Recognition

   Maladaptive Behavior: Difficulty in adaptively recognizing and responding to proprioceptive and/or vibratory stimuli. This can characterize the catatonic individual who will maintain static body positions beyond a seemingly tolerable level.

   Dance-Movement Therapy Techniques:

   1. Movement activities involving experience with proprioceptive recognition; such as:
      a. Activities involving the passive movement of the body or body parts followed by the individual's recognition of the movement. (All categories)
      b. While the individual has his eyes closed, ask him to duplicate various positions which the therapist has either placed the individual's body in or has verbally suggested to him. (All categories)
      c. Suggest to the patient to tense and relax various parts of his body isometrically. (All categories)
      d. Activity involving the massaging of an area followed by the individual's recognition of the stimulation. (All categories)
      e. Movement activity involving resistive exercise with the therapist. For example, hold the client's hands and have him

reciprocally push back and forth, gradually taking the arms through a backward and forward motion while increasing the resistance. (All categories)

2. Activities involving experience with vibratory recognition; such as:
   a. Activity involving the use of a drum or other instrument which gives off vibration. Have the individual touch it with various parts of the body followed by the individual's recognition of the stimulation. (All categories)
   b. Place the individual in certain positions designed to produce vibratory coarcation of muscle bodies. After a period of time, have the individual experience these vibrations and suggest to him that he allow these motions to encompass his whole body in a unified flow. (Neurotics)

Related elements: One-to-one or parallel group; egocentric, object dependent, or object-ambivalent relationship with therapist.

2. Kinesthetic Discrimination

Maladaptive Behavior: Difficulty in adaptively discriminating or localizing proprioceptively and/or vibratorally stimulated body parts; e.g., someone who can't differentiate between his arm moving up or down.

Dance-Movement Therapy Techniques:

Movement activities involving identification of the area of the body and quality of movement based on proprioceptive and/or vibratory stimulations. For example, the therapist may take the person's arm and randomly press it gently and firmly back into the shoulder joint. The individual is asked to verbalize whether the stimulus was gentle or firm. This may of course be graded in difficulty; i.e., more subtle discriminations. (All categories, particularly the blind or organically impaired)

Related elements: One-to-one or parallel group; object-dependent relationship with therapist.

3. Kinesthetic Retention and Recall

Maladaptive Behavior: Inability to hold in memory and duplicate proprioceptive and/or vibratory stimulations.

Dance-Movement Therapy Techniques:

Movement of the body either passively by the therapist or via visual iconic imitation of the therapist's movements followed, after a gradable period of time, by the repetition of the movement by the individual. The movement may be as simple as a gesture or as complicated as a modern dance for a recital. (All categories)

Related elements: Iconic and/or enactive levels of cognition; parallel, task, or egocentric cooperative group; hobby or occupational search such as with a dance club; semi-autonomous chumship, or autonomous relationship with therapist.

## VESTIBULAR PERCEPTUAL LEVELS OF ORGANIZATION[78]

As with the kinesthetic systems, adequate vestibular perception is needed in order to move in a functional, purposeful manner. Without the vestibular apparatus, an individual would be incapable of balancing. He would walk as if in a drunken stupor. No child could possibly begin to be aware of his body without the aid of this sense and its integration with other sense systems such as those mentioned in previous sections. Likewise, an individual in a state of depersonalization can demonstrate a negation of his body which in turn affects the vestibular mechanisms producing a seemingly infantile state.[79] As described by Butter, the functions of the vestibular organs located in the inner ear are as follows:

"The semi-circular canals contain receptors which respond to rotary acceleration of the head, while receptors in the utricle respond to gravitational forces on the head and to linear acceleration. Nerve fibers innervating sensory cells of the vestibular organs travel to the medulla and synapse upon neurons which go to centers controlling eye muscles and neurons in the spinal cord controlling body movement for appropriate postural reactions."[80]

### Vestibular Perceptual Levels of Organization

1. Vestibular Recognition

   This involves the ability to sense vestibular stimulation. Recognition may take the form of a motor reaction such as righting oneself.

2. Vestibular Discrimination

   This involves the capacity to discriminate various vestibular stimulations.

78. The use of the vestibular apparatus in regression in the service of the ego will be discussed later.

79. Schilder, *op. cit.*, p. 167.

80. Charles Butter, *Neuropsychology: The Study of Brain and Behavior* (Belmont: Brooks/Cole Publishing, 1968), p. 108.

3. Vestibular Retention and Recall

This level involves the ability to hold in memory the vestibular stimulation and to duplicate it by reconstructing the movement pattern which produced it, as well as the ability to hold in memory postural positions which reestablished equilibrium.

## Related Maladaptive Behavior with Suggested Methods and Techniques for Dance-Movement Therapy

1. Vestibular Recognition

Maladaptive Behavior: Difficulty in adaptively "catching" self or falling when individual loses balance. This could characterize a person who has so completely depersonalized, who wants to cut himself off from reality to such an extent, that he has tried to cut off body sense systems. (To acknowledge the properties of equilibrium means also to be faced with attending to gravity and to feel "grounded" in reality.)

Dance-Movement Therapy Techniques:

1. Movement activities involving the production of vestibular stimulation—such activities as twirling, rolling, swinging, and other movements which cause body imbalance. Activities such as these serve to reintroduce an individual to his body. (All categories)
2. Passive movement activities involving the production of vestibular stimulation by the therapist, such as tilting of the individual. (All categories) (See Figure III.22.)
3. Movement activities involving the use of objects which facilitate vestibular stimulation such as the use of a trampoline, balance boards, and/or tilt boards. (All categories) (See Figure III.23.)

   Related elements: One-to-one parallel group, egocentric, object-dependent, or object ambivalent relationship with therapist; kinesthetic recognition; gravitational efforts.

2. Vestibular Discrimination

Maladaptive Behavior: Difficulty in adaptively discriminating diverse vestibular stimulation. This can characterize an individual who continuously overreacts by making over-compensating adjustments with each step out of an unrealistic fear of falling.

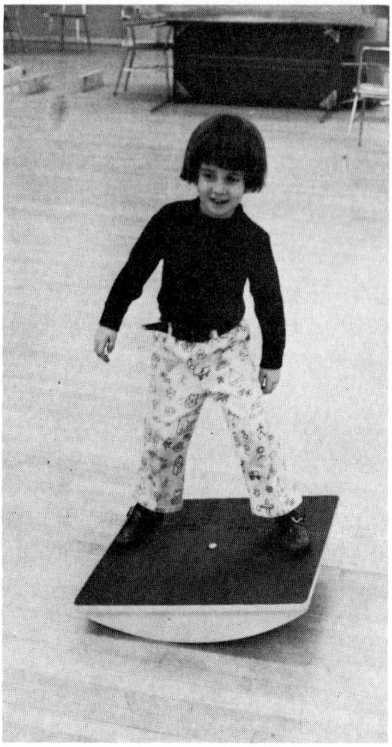

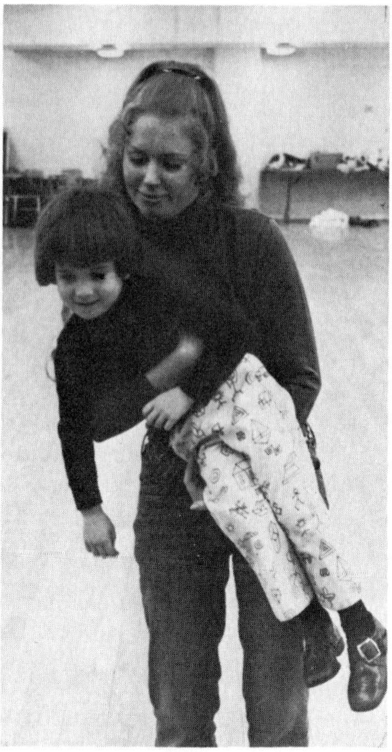

Vestibular stimulation

**Figure III.22.** **Figure III.23.**

Dance-Movement Therapy Techniques:

1. Passive and/or active movement activities involving the discrimination among various vestibular stimulations, e.g., tilting slightly, tilting on more of an angle. Movement activities may be graded in difficulty. For example, to facilitate the activity a mirror can be used to aid in discrimination; to increase the difficulty, the eyes may be closed. (All categories)
2. Movement activities which encourage the exploration of the fear of falling often associated with fears of experiencing unconscious impulses. Pile large foam pillows or mattresses. Start by having the person or group sit on them carefully. Then gradually grade the experience so that they eventually run with abandonment and fall on the pillows. (All categories)

   Related elements: One-to-one or parallel group; object-dependent or object-ambivalent relationship with the therapist; kinesthetic discrimination; gravitational efforts.

3. Vestibular Retention and Recall

   Maladaptive Behavior: Inability to recall the movement pattern which produced a particular vestibular stimulation, and/or inability to recall positions which allowed for the resumption of balance, such as with a child who had difficulty remembering how to catch his balance when pushed backward.

   Dance-Movement Therapy Techniques:

   1. Activity involving movement of the body, either actively or passively, which causes momentary imbalance followed by the individual regaining balance. This is proceeded, after a gradable period of time, by the repetition of the movement of the individual with emphasis on the postural positions used to regain balance. This can be done with the use of ballet positions, or as a game in which the goal is to maintain one's balance during various locomotor activities such as hopping or one and two-legged jumping. (All categories)
   2. Duplicating of activities incorporating the use of fantasy environments such as a tightrope, or a boat on a stormy sea. (All categories)

      Related elements: Iconic and/or enactive level of cognition, parallel group, semi-autonomous or chumship relationship with therapist.

## COGNITIVE REPRESENTATION LEVELS OF ORGANIZATION

Cognition can be defined as the process through which sensory perceptions are appropriately organized such that objects and events are perceived in accordance with one's cultural group. (Mosey, Ruesch, Flavell) It is, in other words, the organization of stimuli with related thought concerning that perception.

Cognitive processes then entail all mental processes concerned with knowing. One of these is the way in which perceptual-motor constructs are remembered. Without this function, no individual could benefit from experience, for each situation would be treated as unique. Its importance is obvious in the integration of adaptive behavior. A movement therapist should, therefore, be aware of the representative level at which his client is functioning in order to insure the full organization of the desired components. If he is facilitating on a higher plane than the individual is capable of comprehending, the session will prove to be frustrating and purposeless. Through acknowledging the cognitive ability of the patient, the therapist may begin to aid him in the integration of higher levels of representation.

## Cognitive Representation Levels of Organization[81]

1. Enactive Cognition

   This level involves the capacity to remember and reproduce a movement response through the use of physical perceptions of the movement pattern as cues. This area also relates to one of the basic principles of dance-movement therapy which recognizes that the most fundamental level of organizing and integrating developmental phases is via enactive cognition and representation. The field further contends that a "talking cure" is insufficient, that the individual's memory entails first a physical body memory and secondarily a language abstract memory. It therefore behooves the clinician to work with the whole person's memory and way of learning and organizing, and that *includes* body-felt experience.

2. Iconic-Imitative Cognition

   This level involves the ability to remember and reproduce a movement response through the use of separate pictorial images or a continuous series of images as cues.

3. Abstract Cognition

   This level involves the ability to remember and reproduce a movement response through the use of concepts, such as verbilization or dance notation as cues.

## Related Maladaptive Behavior with Suggested Methods and Techniques for Dance-Movement Therapy

1. Enactive Cognition

   Maladaptive Behavior: Inability or difficulty in adaptively remembering and/or duplicating the movement response when experienced at an enactive level. For example, an individual who is unable to deeply experience being physically cared for due to early maternal deprivation.

   Dance-Movement Therapy Techniques:

   1. Activities involving the remembering and reproduction of a movement response through the use of enactive physical care. For example, the therapist within an idealized transference, holds and rocks the individual. (All categories)

81. Concepts evolved from Mosey.

2. Passive and active movement exercises (Feldenkrais, Alexander) which assists an individual in becoming aware of and unlearning self-destructive (maladaptive) movement patterns. (All categories)

   Related elements: Kinesthetic retention and recall; vestibular retention and recall; egocentric, object-dependent, or object-ambivalent relationship with therapist.

2. Iconic-Imitative Cognition

   Maladaptive Behavior: Unable to adaptively imitate movements or duplicate movement from pictures. For example, the person cannot imitate the movement of the dance therapist or other group members.

   Dance-Movement Therapy Techniques:

   1. Movement activities involving the use of remembering stimuli in terms of separate pictorial images. For example, the therapist may position himself in one or more postures such as a stance emphasizing presentation of self or communicative asking or giving which the patient views, after which the individual is asked to duplicate it. (All categories, particularly the organically impaired)
   2. Movement activities involving the mirroring of another's movements. This can be graded in complexity. For example, the therapist and client face each other, and first move holding hands (enactive), gradually diminishing physical contact. (All categories)
   3. Movement activities involving the individual duplicating a movement that he has just viewed. This can be a gesture or a sequence. The therapist may wish to make use of gestures, dynamics, and shape which the person utilizes in his own movement signature. (All categories)
   4. Movement activities involving the duplication of movements of non-human objects. For example, the therapist could drop a scarf to the ground and suggest that the group simulate the quality. (All categories)

      Related elements: Parallel, task, egocentric and cooperative group; object-ambivalent or semi-autonomous relationship with therapist.

3. Abstract Cognition

   Maladaptive Behavior: Inability or difficulty in adaptively remembering and/or reproducing a movement through the use of concepts.

For example, someone may be able to bend over after he has seen the therapist do it, but be unable to reproduce the pattern if only given the verbal cue of "Bend over." This might also characterize a person who has difficulty translating labanotation into movement even after he has been taught what the symbols mean. This same person may be able to quickly pick up and learn a dance if he is shown the pattern.

Dance-Movement Therapy Techniques:

1. Movement activities involving the use of verbalization as a stimulus for the pattern. For example, making use of movements which the therapist has seen the person do, he might suggest some of these verbally to the person. This can be graded by first telling the person and showing the pattern simultaneously several times so that an association is made, followed by the verbal cue alone. (All categories when age-appropriate)
2. Dance activities involving the use of a verbal imagery and abstract concepts; for example, asking the individual or group to move in response to words such as freedom, anger, joy, sadness, etc. (All categories when age-appropriate)
3. Movement activities involving the use of a notational system. For example, have an individual or group make up a dance, notate it in some written fashion, and then, after a period of time, reproduce the work from the notation. (All categories when age appropriate)
4. Charades. (All categories)

   Related elements: Use of play-work: hobby or occupational search; task or egocentric-cooperative group; semi-autonomous, chumship, or autonomous relationship with therapist.

## THOUGHT PROCESS LEVELS OF ORGANIZATION

One of the most important areas in which movement therapists can play a major role is the evolving of an individual from a solely primary process to that of reality-stressed secondary process orientation. Since the primary process level is often characterized by symbolic nonverbal behavior (an area which is often foreign to the verbal-oriented psychiatrist or psychologist), the dance therapist may be one of the few on the team who can actively involve the patient in psychotherapy. Because of his specialized training in body language, he may understand what the patient is trying to say and thus provide a primary bond for the development of a needed pre-oediple transference.[82] The movement therapist, due to the ability of creative body movement to tap into the unconscious more directly than other, more traditional verbal psychotherapies (Zwerling), is also effective in working with the individual who has no access into his unconscious and is locked into secondary process. Movement is a basic universal bridge between both thought processes.

### Thought Process Levels of Organization

1. Primary Process Thought

   This level involves the maintenance of knowledge and thought processes on an unconscious level. Archetypal[83] and idiosyncratic symbolism prevail along with an anaclytic narcissistic relationship with the environment and disregard for properties of weight, space, and time. The individual is said to be guided by the pleasure principle. (Freud)[84]

2. Secondary Process Thought

   This level involves the maturation of cognition and is used in the ordering of conscious mental content. The individual is able to differentiate himself from his environment and relate to persons in a nondependent manner. Awareness and functional use of the qualities of weight, space, and time is also characteristic of this level. The individual is now also guided by the reality principle. (Freud)

3. Tertiary Process[85]

   This stage involves the conscious awareness and discrimination among material which is derived solely from the unconscious, that which is partially from the unconscious and partially from the conscious level, and/or that which is solely from the conscious level. Along with the integration of this skill comes creativity in its purest form which is unincumbered by the need to perpetuate neurotic or psychotic movements. At this level the "bridge"[86] between the conscious and the unconscious is open, allowing free flow of psychic energy.

82. At this basic level it is also sometimes necessary to utilize one's own unconscious in order to better understand and relate to an individual utilizing primary process thought. In this way the therapist can more accurately sense the appropriate length of time needed by the patient to understand this strange "underworld" of repressed symbolized material. (Sullivan, Rosen, Searles, Laing, Sesahahye)

83. Carl Jung, *Man and His Symbols* (New York:Doubleday & Co., 1964).

84. Mosey, *op. cit.*, p. 15.

85. Ann Mosey, *Three Frames of Reference for Mental Health* (Charles Block, 1970), p. 51.

86. Jung, *op. cit.*

4. Quaternary Process

   This level entails the awareness and discrimination among thought which emanates from secondary process, thought which is primary process emerging from the personal unconscious, and thought which is of an archetypal universal symbolic nature from the collective unconscious. From a Jungian developmental point of view, in the middle years, the Self replaces the ego in primacy, allowing for richer fuller contact with the transpersonal. (See Chapter VII, Relationship of the Transpersonal to a Developmental Theory of Dance-Movement Therapy, and also Ego Psychology, Jungian Analytic Psychology and Related Developmental Constellations in the Appendix for further delineation.)

### Related Maladaptive Behavior with Suggested Methods and Techniques for Dance-Movement Therapy

1. Primary Process

   Maladaptive Behavior: Predominance of solely neutral flow; the individual is literally drowning in their unconscious.

   Dance-Movement Therapy Techniques:

   1. Movement activities involving use of symbolic imagery and movements; such as a movement sequence which involves the individual going into and coming out of a body of water and experiencing grounding himself. (All categories)
   2. Movement activities which help the individual journey into his unconscious primary process world. (Sullivan, Fromm-Reichman, Searles, Jung, and Laing) The individual himself is often the best catalyst, as he lives in the symbiotic world. These symbolic processes can be enacted or reenacted in movement dramas. Each character as well as meaningful (symbolically charged) objects should be played out by the individual. (Gestalt) (Adults, neurotics, children)

      Related elements: Flow of breath; symmetrical shape and tension flow; flow rhythms, one-to-one group; egocentric relationship to therapist.

2. Secondary Process

   A. Maladaptive Behavior: Inadaptive use of archetypal and idiosyncratic symbols in lieu of reality-oriented secondary process thought. For example, bizarre gestures, mannerisms, and possible verbalizations which are not understood by one's cultural group due to their unconscious origin.

Dance-Movement Therapy Techniques:

1. Activities stressing the use of reality-oriented movement patterns with reflective verbalization. The therapist may wish to involve the person in very simple activities such as catching a ball, standing, sitting, and sensing his body in relationship to general environmental variables.
2. Activities involving the establishment of eye contact; such as, a game in which the therapist and child take turns trying to look in the other's eyes while the other tries to avoid contact. (All categories)

B. Maladaptive Behavior: Difficulty or lack of adaptive functional use of weight, space, and time as demonstrated by a poor effort-shape repertoire.

Dance-Movement Therapy Techniques:

Activities involving the awareness and functional integration of movements requiring the use of qualities of weight, space, and time (use of all pre-efforts, directional shape, effort, and shaping) within the individual's idiosyncratic behavioral repertoire (See Effort-Shape areas for further clarification and illustration.) (All categories)

C. Maladaptive Behavior: Predominance of nonverbal behavior; i.e., does not verbalize when appropriate.

Dance-Movement Therapy Techniques:

Refer to Flow of Breath and Symmetrical Shape Flow. (All categories)

Related elements: Perceptual stimulation, Effort-Shape variables; Flow of Breath; Object-ambivalent relationship with therapist; one-to-one, parallel, or task group.

3. Tertiary Process

A. Maladaptive Behavior: Inability to discriminate primary process thought from secondary process thought.

Dance-Movement Therapy Techniques:

Activities involving exploration and discrimination between movements which are reality-oriented involving secondary process thought and movements which are symbolic in nature involving primary process thought. For example, involving a group in a fantasy-movement drama followed by a movement game with the end of the session devoted to talking about the felt differences. (All categories)

B. Maladaptive Behavior: Ego defensive structure does not allow access to the unconscious; e.g. no recollection of dreams or inability to free associate verbally, minimal pure tension flow rhythms, blocked shape flow and flow of breath, dominence of efforts and shaping to the exclusion of flow fluctations.

Dance-Movement Therapy Techniques:

Non-directed authentic movement improvisations as free association or active imagination. This is a process in which the individual places himself in a state of active receptivity (yin state) and allows any movement with its associated images and emotions to emerge, unedited by the ego. Whitehouse describes this as an experience of "being moved."[87] (Individuals with existing egos)

Related elements: Use of creative improvisations, parallel, task or egocentric-cooperative group; semi-autonomous, chumship, or autonomous relationship with therapist.

4. Quaternary Process

A. Maladaptive Behavior: Inability to contact archetypal core of complexes due to the overriding personal unconscious material inhibiting connection.

Dance-Movement Therapy Techniques:

1. Developmental movement therapy which serves to identify, explore, and integrate those personal relationships which inhibit connection to the archetypal. Encouragement of positive transference once negative expressions with significant others have been fully explored will often facilitate what Jung called a "transpersonal counterpoint" in which energy cathected to the therapist can shift to the archetypal.[88] (Individuals capable of forming a working alliance [Greenson])
2. Directed imagery movement improvisations which stress connection to the spiritual and archetypal. Personifications such as Demeter/earth mother, Kali, Zeus, sun god, moon, trickster, witch, puer, puella, guru, senex, dragon, Eros, monster-beast,

87. Mary Whitehouse, "C. G. Jung and Dance Therapy: Two Major Principles;" Bernstein, Ed., *Eight Theoretical Approaches in Dance-Movement Therapy* (Dubuque: Kendall/Hunt Pub., 1979) p. 57–58.

88. Penny Bernstein, "The Inter-Intra-Transpersonal Matrix in Jungian Dance Therapy," paper presented at the American Dance Therapy Association, Los Angeles, 1980.

tree, snake, fool, Mercury, Janus, Holy Spirit, devil, gold, butterfly, earth, air, fire, water, etc., can be enacted or related to. (All categories)

B. Maladaptive Behavior:Inability to experience the individual's life in relation to a mythologem, personal quest or journey.

Dance-Movement Therapy Techniques:

1. Movement improvisations which explore an individual's personification of alchemy. (Alchemy is viewed here as a symbolic process which attempts to make gold out of baser materials. In a individual's life this is translated to his quest for individuation and enlightenment, e.g., the quest for the Holy Grail.)

   The four stages are:

   a. Black: awareness of shadow, unintegrated parts, latent forces, and guilt.
   b. White: Exploration, minor work, and beginning changes
   c. Red: Passion, emotionl catharsis.
   d. Gold: Integration, illumination, connection to the transpersonal.[89] (All categories)

2. Movement dramas which are enactments of stories, myths, and fairytales which the individual identifies as paraleling his own personal mythic journeys.[90] For example, a woman might relate to the classic Demeter-Persephone myth or other women's initiation rites in which a *hieros gamos* or sacred marriage occurs such as with the vestal virgins in the greek temples. Waiting, accepting, surrendering, ripening, transforming are all part of the process. The goal is to become a virgin i.e. a woman, free, not bound by personal desires or egotism, able to experience her own instinct without the justification of a man's love—to be "one-in-herself" (Harding, Hall). (All categories)

3. Movement dramas which stress the individual's enactment of his own mythic journey through life. (See Case Studies:Mark.) (All categories)

4. Use of art activities such as the Jungian sand tray[91] or the drawing of one's life history followed by a moving out of the pictoral representations. (All categories)

   Related elements:Aging process and dying ritual process.

89. J. E. Cirlot, *A Dictionary of Symbols (New York: Philosophical Library, 1978).*

90. *Ibid.*

91. Penny Bernstein, "A Mythic Quest:Jungian Movement Therapy with the Psychosomatic Client" *American Journal of Dance Therapy,* vol. 3, no. 2, 1980.

## PLAY-WORK LEVELS OF ORGANIZATION[92]

Finally, movement, and more specifically dance as an art form, may be utilized in organizing skills needed for leisure activities as well as for an occupation.

Before discussing the levels of this area, it should be made clear that the use of dance in this manner is generally applicable to only a small portion of patients, if any at all. This area is utilized on an adult level *only* if the individual has an interest in movement beyond its purely therapeutic benefits, and only *after* he has partaken of all that Dance Therapy may offer him. Because of the confusing nature of coupling therapeutic dance with social dance or dance as an art form, these two very separate areas should never be combined. It is extremely perplexing to a patient if he perceives the session as solely "social dancing" or a "dance technique class" and the leader intends to do "Movement Therapy." For children and adolescents, however, the use of play as transitional space is richly fertile (Winnicott).

This final area is therefore seen as a prelude to leaving the hospital or as a weaning process by the therapist, and it should be utilized only after the individual has organized all the major adaptive patterns he needs in order to function adequately in his environment.

### Play-Work Levels of Organization

1. Dance as a Hobby

   This level involves the ability to make use of dance as an expressive creative tool for leisure time. This entails being able to utilize dance extemporaneously. The body, as a dancer's tool, should be sufficiently conditioned and exercised so as to insure the artistic quality needed.

2. Dance as an Occupation

   This level involves the acquisition of the needed dance skills for the particular dance form of choice. Choreography, entailing the ability to creatively problem-solve, may or may not be integrated at this time.

### Related Maladaptive Behavior with Suggested Method and Techniques for Dance Movement Therapy

1. Dance as a Hobby

   A. Maladaptive Behavior: Body insufficiently conditioned. This could be characterized by an individual who is unable to endure more than a few minutes of dancing without exhaustion.

92. Adapted from Mosey.

Dance-Movement Therapy Techniques:

Movement activities on a regular schedule designed to stretch; strengthen; increase range of motion; and work on placement, dance technique, and/or endurance. These sessions can be styled after traditional dance classes. (All categories)

B. Maladaptive Behavior: Difficulty in improvisational dance. This can characterize a person who has always directed his life according to various authority figures (e.g., parents, teachers, therapists) and has a great deal of difficulty moving in a spontaneous creative manner.

Dance-Movement Therapy Techniques:

Movement activities involving dancing extemporaneously for self-expression or in response to cues such as music and/or a selected image. This can be graded from gesture to dance. (All categories)

Related elements: Semi-autonomous or autonomous relationship with therapist, aging, ritual process, all levels of all other areas.

2. Dance as an Occupation

Maladaptive Behavior: Difficulty in creative problem-solving; such as someone who is unable to choreograph a dance.

Dance-Movement Therapy Techniques:

1. Choreographic problem-solving activities. For example, suggest to the individual (or group) that he choreograph his personal life journey. (All categories)
2. The production of a recital to be performed for the hospital or the community by the individual or group. (All categories)

   Related elements: Semi-autonomous or autonomous relationship with therapist; all levels of other areas.

# CHAPTER IV

# Regression in the Service of the Ego

"The general assumption is that under certain conditions the ego regulates regression, and that the integrative functions of the ego include voluntary and temporary withdrawal of cathexis." Kris[1]

Occasionally it is necessary to make use of movement techniques of regression in order to facilitate the therapeutic process in the learning of adaptive levels of organization. This procedure is indicated with the individual who has fixated at the pre-genital level of development due to inadequate integration or organization of a level or phase. (Freud, Whiting[2]) Although the person continues to evolve into maturity, the faulty learning at an earlier age may predispose him to a behavior disorder when stressful situations arise.[3] (Erikson, 1965, pp. 95–96)

Freud writes on this subject:

"Most closely studied in analysis is temporal regression in drive and libido development. What is affected here, on the one hand, is the choice of objects and the relations to them, with consequent returns to those of earliest significance and the most infantile expressions of dependence. On the other hand, the drive organization may be affected as a whole, and reverting to earlier pregenital levels and to the aggressive manifestations coordinated with them may be brought about. Regression in this respect is considered as based on a specific characteristic of drive development, namely, on the fact that while libido and aggression move forward from one level to the next and cathect the objects which serve satisfaction on each stage, no station on the way is every fully outgrown, as it is on the organic side. While one part of the drive energy is on a forward course, other portions of it, of varying quantity, remain behind, tied to earlier aims and objects, and create the so-called *fixation points* (to autoerotism and narcissism, to the stages of the infant-mother relationship, preoedipal and oedipal dependency, to oral pleasures and oral sadism, to anal-sadistic or passive-masochistic attitudes, phallic masturbation,

1. Ernst Kris, *Psychoanalytic Explorations in Art* (New York: Schocken Books, 1967), p. 312.

2. John Whiting and Irwin Child, *Child Training and Personality* (New Haven: Yale University Press, 1953).

3. These so-called stressful situations generally bear some relationship to the initial level and etiology of the inadequate development.

exhibitionism, egocentricity, etc.). Fixation points may be caused by any type of traumatic experience, by either excessive frustration or excessive gratification on any of these levels, and may exist with different degrees of awareness and consciousness or repression and unconsciousness attached to them. For the developmental outcome this is less important than the fact that for whatever cause and in either state they have the function of binding and retaining drive energies and that thereby they impoverish later drive functioning and object relations.

"Fixations and regressions have always been regarded as interdependent. By virtue of their very existence and according to the measure of libido and aggression with which they are cathected, the fixation points exert a constant retrograde pull on drive activity, an attraction which makes itself felt during all early development and in maturity."

Referrals generally occur after a "stressful situation" has transpired; however, more and more, movement therapists have been acting on a prophylactic level, treating the so-called normal neurotic. Whether the therapist comes in contact with his client before or after a crisis event is not as important a factor as is the therapist's ability to recognize an individual with an unstable foundation.

The role of the movement therapist, then, is to (1) observe the movement repertoire of the individual, (2) determine at what level inadequate learning occurred, (3) with the establishment of a developmentally appropriate transference assist the individual in his natural regression process to the initial level of malfunction (fixation point), (4) explore through movement re-enactments traumatic experiences or prototypical situations which resulted in the fixation, and (5) utilize all the necessary components from the appropriate levels of organization to provide an environment in which the individual can integrate those adaptive patterns that are needed in a functioning movement repertoire. This process occurs as a natural progression in any depth movement therapy. Thus the client's own idiosyncratic timing becomes the guiding force.

There are basic crucial components which are needed in order for an adaptive pattern to be fully integrated or organized. Therefore, a "total movement activity" creating a "total environment" is required. It should also be noted that by "total environment" the internal as well as external environment of a client is taken into consideration. It is up to the therapist to facilitate the appropriate internal setting for the organization of the somatopsychic components. It is this last area in which regression is most needed; i.e., as a tool to bring about the appropriate psychic state. An individual cannot be expected to integrate appropriately the egocentric level of the dyadic constellation if he is attempting to function on an emotional level which required autonomous interactions with the therapist.

There are those who dispute the use of regression, stating that even though an individual is not functioning on a totally integrated manner, he nonetheless can get by. Some even feel that anyone who involves himself in such a process would demonstrate that his ego boundaries are weak and ineffectual. To some, the behavior of this person would be labeled more maladaptive than that of another who rigidly refuses this process in spite of his need. However, regression to the fixation point has been inherent in every depth psychoanalysis. Regression in the service of the ego is evidence of a "strong," not a "weak" ego, it is evidence of an ego which has the capacity to regress in part while the depth and duration of the regression are controlled by the ego as a whole (Gill, Brenman, Mosey, Laing, Klein, Freud).

## MOVEMENT AS A REGRESSIVE TOOL

Movement for obvious reasons lends itself beautifully to a regressive process. Meerloo states, "The sharing of gestures, movements, and feelings brings man back to the blessed state of dependency and togetherness which he had to relinquish in the process of growing up and becoming an individual." He goes on to point out the early biologic roots of dance, stating that in his clinical practice he has experienced dance students who used their "dance aspirations as a means to return unobstrusively to frustrated desperate moods carried over from childhood." He sites the use of dancing to rock music as a regressive tool of the young. Paul Schilder has often mentioned that through movement comes a departure from the typically rigid state to a more loosened and dissolved state such that the body is then able to return to one of the primary attitudes.[4]

Movement as a vehicle for regression has particular relevance when working with individuals whose fixation points are at a preverbal level. Those individuals with narcissictic personality disorders are in part functioning within the symbiotic phase of development. Thus the maladaptive environment occurred at a time when verbal language was unavailable. Quite often these individuals cannot verbally articulate or associate to these pre-verbal wounds as they were received via the sensori-motor pathways of the limbic system of the brain. Cortical functioning with all its sophistication had not sufficiently developed. Movement rather than verbalization becomes the vehicle of choice not only to facilitate the regression but for the re-experiencing of the narcissistic wounds. Likewise the organization and reinternalization of a narcissistic mirror or idealizing transference can not fully take place on a verbal level since this process normally takes place non-verbally. Holding with attunement to the individual can provide prototypical schemata and build up enactively experienced memories which will provide the needed foundation for self-esteem, self-confidence, empathy, creativity, and depth (Kohut).

4. Schilder, *op. cit.*, p. 207.

The psycho-physiological process of regression may be described as a sensing that the body ego is slipping away from one's ego control. Distal extremities go before medial, caudal before cephalo, and the less sensitive, less charged areas before the erotogenic zones, areas laden with libidinal energy.[5] Disassociation often sets in with the loss of coordinated functioning. A predominance of more primitive drive-discharged rhythms appear in their pure form; urethral, then anal, then oral rhythms take over the body. Utilization of effort-shape variables is virtually non-existent, only tension flow and shape flow remain.

## GENERAL MODES OF REGRESSION

A regressive movement can be initiated in any one of a number of ways. Increased strength of instinctual impulses, change in the apparatus available to the ego for adaptive functioning, and/or alteration in the external situation are three main avenues that will be discussed in this chapter.[6]

I. Increased Strength of Instinctual Impulses—is the most widely used among professionals in Movement Therapy. Some examples of this type are:

1. Anal Level Regression
    a. Movement activity involving a temper tantrum state. While lying prone on a mat or bed, the individual is asked to kick the mat with the back of each leg, alternating legs; the arms with both hands making fists should also be hitting the mat, alternating as well.[7] If the exercise is physically integrated, the head will begin to move from side to side in rhythm with the rest of the body movement. (Lowen) (See Figure III–7.)
    b. Hitting a pillow, bed, or punching bag with gesture-posture merging while yelling, "no," "I won't," or "leave me alone."
2. Oral Level Regression
    a. Movement activities involving the person lying prone on a mat with his arms extended in the air. The person is then asked to call for his mother (or father) in the manner in which he would have as a child. (Lowen) (See Figure IV–1.)

5. Paul Federn, M.D., *Ego Psychology and the Psychosis* (New York: Basic Books, 1952), p. 29.

6. Jesse Gorden, ed., *Handbook of Clinical and Experimental Hypnosis* (New York: MacMillan Co., 1967), p. 294.

7. It is important to note here that arms and legs should also be in opposition when hitting the mat, e.g., (R) arm (L) leg.

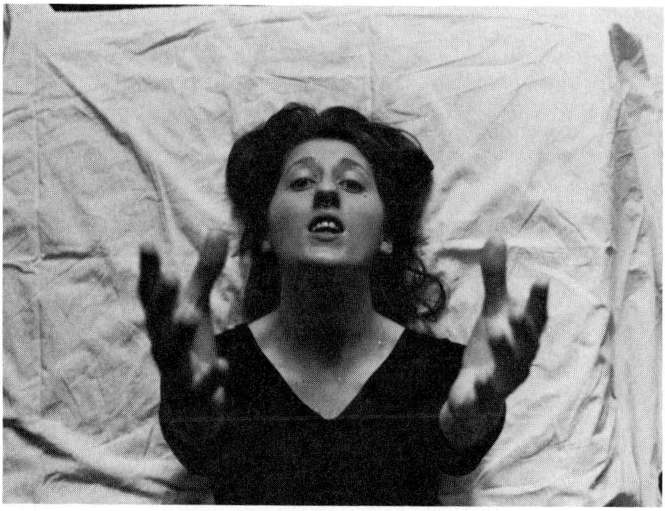

**Figure IV.1.**

b. Movement activities involving the rocking of the individual in a fetal position by another using oral libidinal rhythms while attending to his primal needs (egocentric relationship).

II. Change in the apparatuses available to the ego for adaptive functioning. Sensori-motor is the primary apparatus. Some examples of this type are:

1. Movement activities involving the use of spinning without spotting. Dizziness is often accompanied by regressive depersonalization since both have the same psychic nucleus. (Schilder)
2. Desensitization of the individual through swaddling; eyes are kept closed with a minimum of auditory stimulation. Individual may be rocked in an oral rhythm.
3. Group movement dance using repetitive rhythmic body action of known ritual rhythms used in various cultures.

III. Alteration of the external situation—(It is difficult at best to separate this area from the other two, particularly #II. Techniques are generally a combination of all three with emphasis in different areas.) However, some examples which seem to emphasize this aspect are:

1. In Utero Regression

   Movement activities involving the use of a heated pool. The water can become the warm amniotic fluid of the womb to an individual who is held loosely in a fetal position by another. The eyes should be closed and the ears submerged if at all possible. The movement takes the form of the breath pulse of the individual who is holding the client. A group can also be used, each member holding on to part of the individual's body.

2. Oral Level Regression

   A similar group configuration is the familiar group rock in which one member is picked up prone by the group and rocked at their waist level. Members often hum a lullaby. (See Figure IV–2.)

3. Anal Level Regression

   Large plastic sheeting covers the floor. Finger paints or soap based media are provided for the properly clothed individual or group to finger, foot, and/or body paint. Typically a gradual regression occurs in which painting self and others develops into body smearing and playfulness.

Most other methods are too difficult to separate out and classify in these three areas. One of the most common approaches centers around the sensory regressive technique in which the therapist assunes the role of a verbal facilitator guiding the individual or group back to a primary state. The voice is almost a monotone, hynotic, and follows the breath pattern of the group. Evenness of breath, relaxation of tension, and loosening of ego boundaries producing a merging with the environment is stressed.

### "The Heep"

There are other methods in which the therapist's role is solely that of initiator and observer-care taker. One which may provide assistance in this process in "the heep." It is valuable not only as a regressive technique, but also as a diagnostic tool to determine both the individual and group level of fixation. Its primary use has been with groups, although it can easily be adapted to individual treatment with the involvement of the therapist in a "dyad heep." The verbal stimuli for the group is:

"I would now like you to silently choose a place on the floor and form a clump or a heep such that everyone is touching at least one other member. You may lie, sit, stand—whichever seems most appropriate to you. (Group forms a heep.) Now relax, close your eyes, and get into yourself, and listen to your body. If you feel like moving, do so, whether it is by yourself or with other members of the group. If you feel like maintaining your position throughout this experience, that is o.k. too. There may be times you may feel bored; that too is o.k. Just listen to your body and do what you want to do. I ask

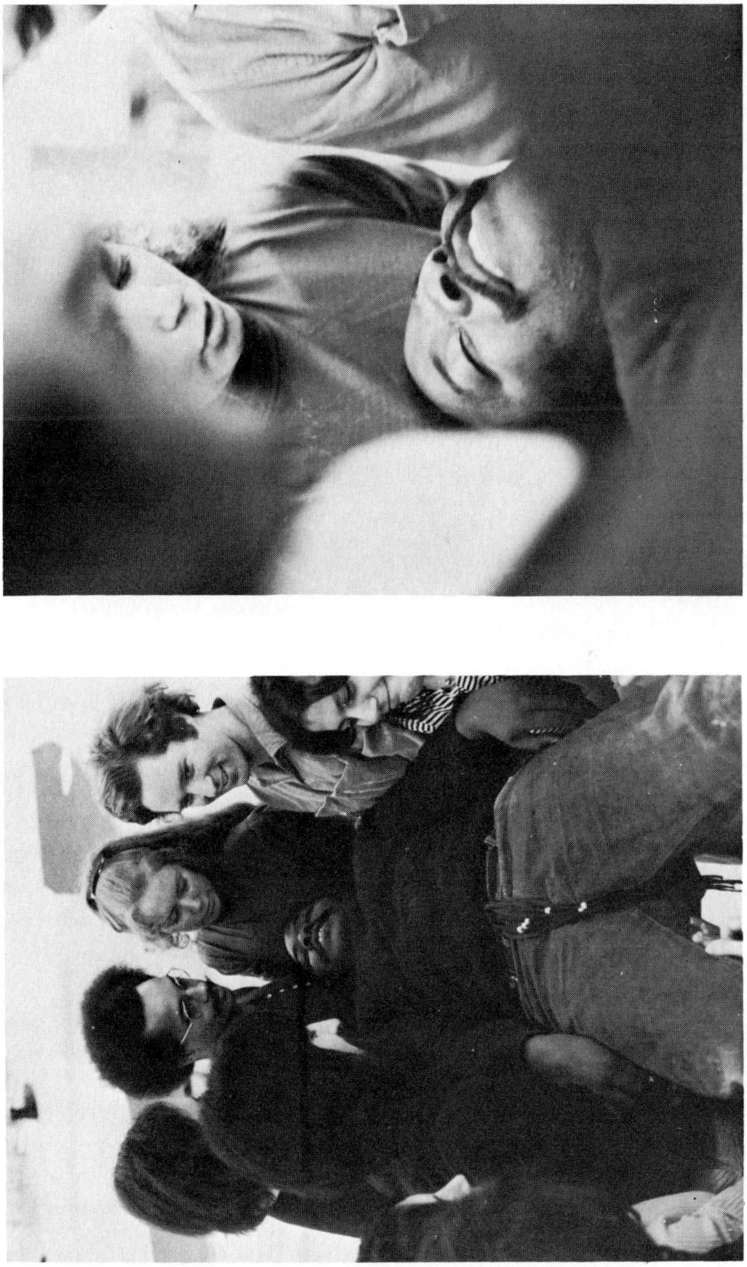

A

B

Figure IV.2.

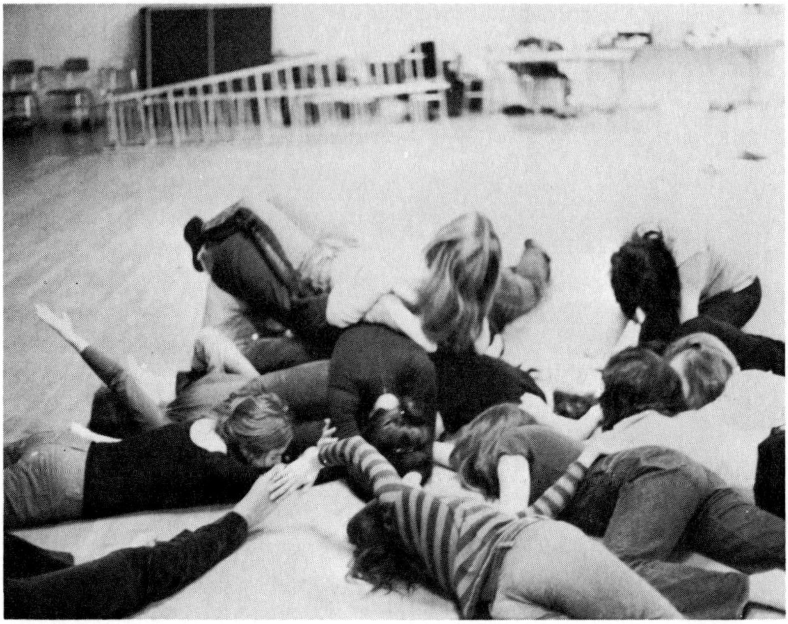

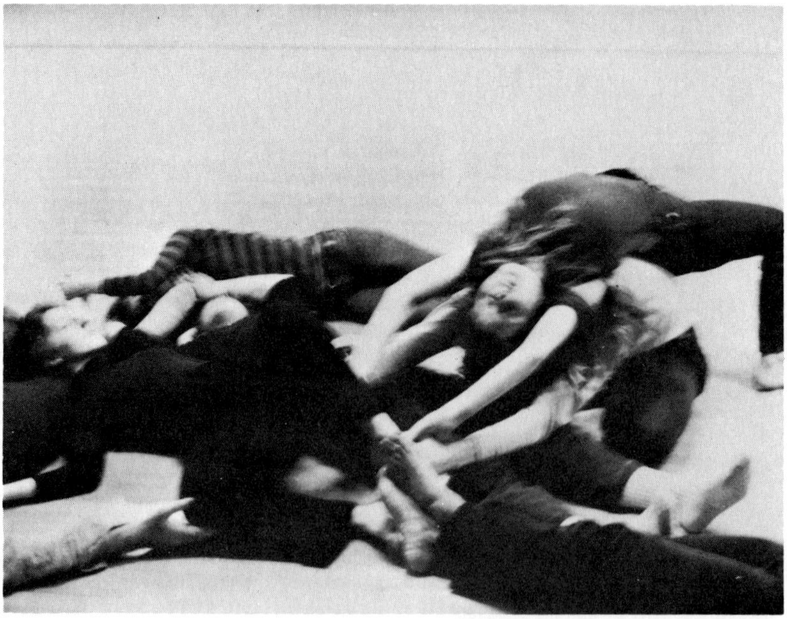

The "Heep"

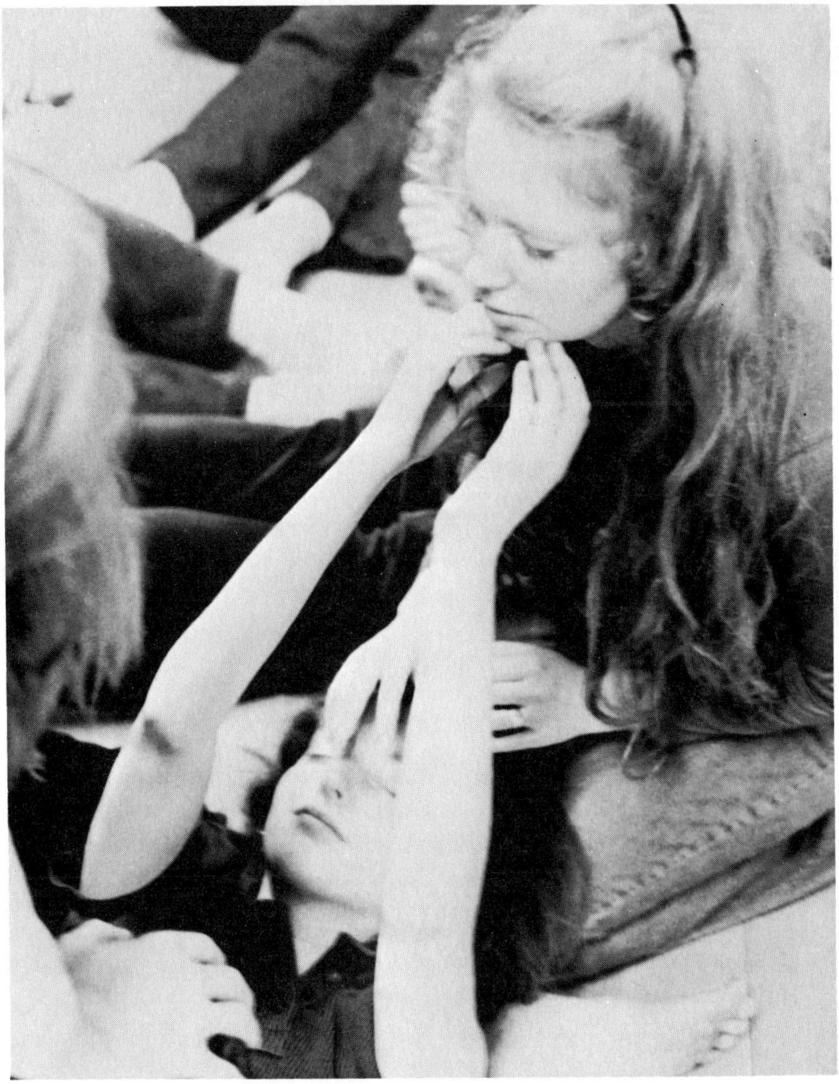

The "Heep" (continued)

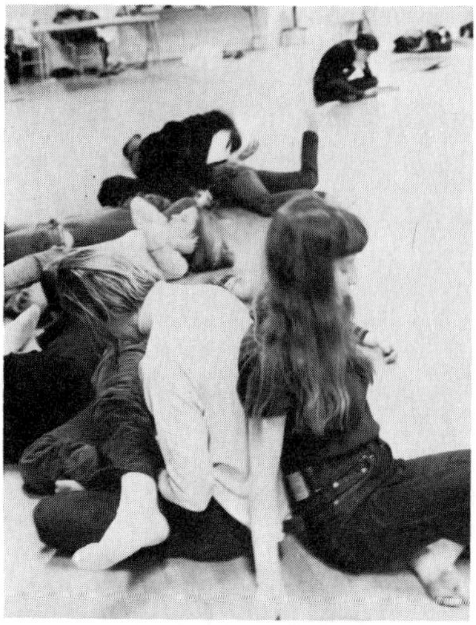

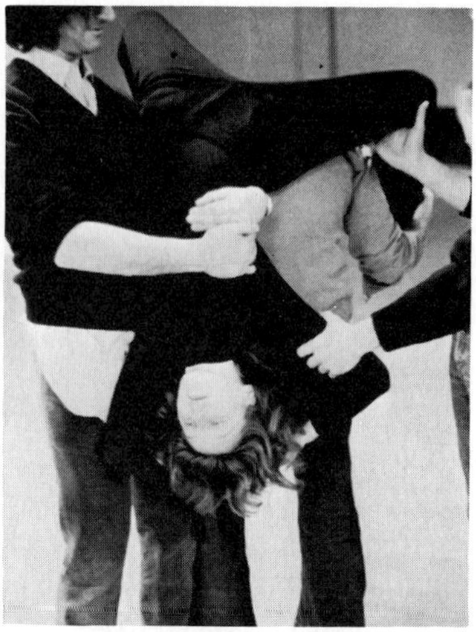

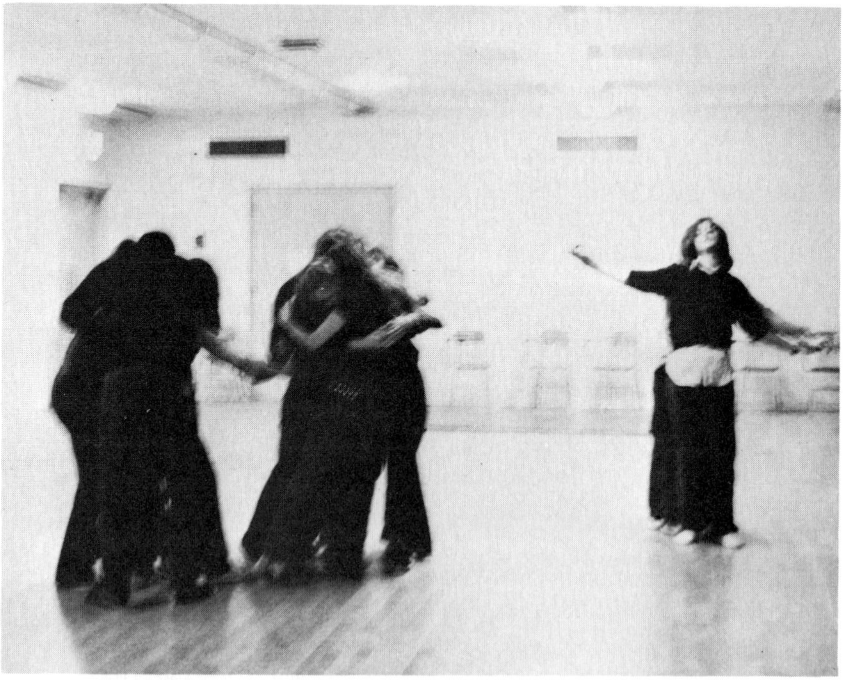

The "Heep" (continued)

only that if you wish to communicate with another that it be on a nonverbal level. This experience will be completed when everyone has stopped moving."

The lights are then dimmed, and music which has little or no dynamic changes—changes which might infringe upon the mood state of an individual—is played. Indian music, Zen meditation music, "white sound," chants, or music from the Impressionist period can be used.

Diagnostically what has been observed is that individuals in this exercise will recapitulate human development, and if there are any holes in integration of adaptive patterns they will fixate at those levels. For example, the observer may see one person move off from the group and rock by himself while another can be seen groping around the group in attempts to find someone who is moving in an oral rhythm, while another is seen continually forcing his own movement patterns on others.

If a group is a truly cohesive and functioning unit, they will be seen moving together in a unified and varying rhythm. They will also eventually be "off the ground" and moving through space. (See pp. 152–153.)

## RECAPITULATION AND SUMMARY

Recapitulation takes place when (1) the level of fixation is ascertained, and (2) the needed primal adaptive levels are integrated or organized. Quite often the recapitulation process is a natural result of the resolution of these primitive conflict areas. In any case, regression is frequently a necessary tool. When it is used not as an escape mechanism but rather "in the service of the ego," it becomes a vehicle in which the movement therapist can assist his client to a stronger, healthier level of functioning.

In summary, it is also important to note that if the therapeutic relationship develops to the extent that a working alliance is formed, the individual will naturally begin to allow regression through movement free associational experiences. In these cases, the client will provide the timing and form of the regression and with the therapist's assistance in verbal processing and in facilitating the environment for the organization of the developmental components, integrate the phase and move to his age-appropriate level of functioning. (See Diane's case study for an example of this process.)

# CHAPTER V

# Somatatization of Symbols

Regardless of physical or psychic state, unconscious symbolic somatatizations may be continuously active in the body attitude and movement repertoire of any person. The symbolic process may take the form of a tense body part, dead spot, pained area, organ dysfunction, body posture, or seemingly unobtrusive gesture or postural movement. The rationale and development of these symbolically charged areas varies among individuals, their experiences, and their predisposition to somatatize symptoms of psychic disfunction. One avenue is through parental and/or peer attitudes toward parts of the body and their functioning. In this case, the body-image equipped with symbolic cathexis evolves through experiencing and integrating the thoughts and actions of those in the environment.

The body is often seen as the "screen" of the ego upon which the individual projects feelings about himself and the world. Illnesses, operations, and accidents are also said to leave permanent psychosomatic tension spots which are laden with symbolism. Generally it is felt, however (particularly in the case of tension areas) that this process is due to conflict directly related to one or more of the functions of a particular part. Lowen states, "The correlation between muscle tensions and inhibition is so exact that one can tell what impulses or feelings are inhibited in a person from a study of his muscular tensions."[1] In other words, the desire to do an act (utilization of solely agonist muscles) is counteracted by fear, guilt, double-bind, etc. (utilization of antagonist muscles as well), thus producing a tense body or body parts. Too much rigidity leads then to compulsiveness around conflict areas. The opposite, too much flaccidity, leads to impulsiveness with possible suicidal ideation[2] (Lowen, Rothstein).

Along with the symbolism placed in body parts, is the symbolic investment of certain movements. Felix Deutsch designed a method of "analytic posturology" which traces and evaluates the symbolism in certain motor behavior.

1. Alexander, M.D., "Breathing, Movement, and Feeling" (reprint, 1965), p. 27.

2. Do not confuse these symptoms with the spasticity caused by CNS dynsfunction or flaccidity caused by muscular or peripheral neuropathic illnesses and trauma.

The symbolic process often carries with it an extra raison d'etre which can be regarded as a somatatized resistance. Tension areas usually produce "dead spots" which aid in the blocking or repression of the conflict areas. Compulsive movements which serve as undoing, compensating, or regressive mechanisms are examples of this phenomenon, as are the pre-efforts as defense mechanisms discussed earlier.

## SOME EXAMPLES OF SYMBOLIC BODY PART INVESTMENT

(Reich, Schilder, Lowen, Allport, Kubie,
Deutsch, Machover, Urban, Christensen)

Eyes

— "windows of the soul"
— felt to reveal inner feelings
—half closed or downward gaze: reluctance to view the world due to possible hostility toward others
—symbolize openings through which the environment can wander in
—incorporative attitudes, one who is afraid of being incorporated
—straining: wanting to see through everything
—tension due to inhibition of peri-occular muscles: desire to hold back crying

Nose

—symbol of sexuality and power strivings
—continuous snorts: primitive aggression
—tension due to fear of breathing in poision, radar, gas, etc., (Paranoidal ideation)
—continuous shallow sniffs: fear of taking in or letting go

Mouth, Teeth, and Jaw

—mouth emphasized; oral eroticism
—tense: refusal to reveal self
—tense: rejection of dependent needs
—teeth clenched: oral aggressiveness
—teeth clenched: biting sarcasm
—tension: inhibition of crying and sadness
—tension: inhibition of anger
—tension: fear of taking anything in, e.g., an expressed thought or feeling of another
—inhibition of biting impulses

Neck and Throat

—hypertonus of neck: displaced genital anxiety
—tension: something "can't be swallowed"

—tension: something or someone who is a "pain in the neck"
—tension: a means of cutting off body emotions which have been in the heart or gut area
—tension: a means of insuring lack of intellectual or conscious awareness of feelings placed in the body, i.e., the head is cut off from his body
—tension: fear of being struck from behind
—tension: fear of screaming out
—tension: fear of losing one's head

Shoulders, Arms, and Hands

—provide strength and power and indicate power strivings
—depressed: an attempt to hold back aggression, holding from striking out
—raised: fear, scared stiff
—Arms are instrumental in:
 "handling" the world
 rejecting others
 reaching out to or pushing away others
 aggressing or defending oneself
 carrying out operations
—tension: fear or guilt over hitting out
—hands: tools for manipulating environment
—weak hands, arms: inadequacy feelings

Chest and Stomach

—pain: suppression of sadness—longing
—queasy: can't stomach something
—tension: repression of sadness
—tension: repression of anger
—conflict between infantile oral craving and super-ego adult rejection

Pelvis and Genitals[3]

—tension and blockage of flow: denial of full sexuality
—tension and blockage of flow: fear of castration

Back

—backache syndrome: on guard, wavering between fight and flight
—tension: inability to mobilize anger to overcome frustration
—lordosis: sexual dysfunction[4]

3. Other parts of the body which protrude such as the nose, foot, etc., may also serve as substitute phallic zones with similar rationales for symbolic investment.

4. Do not confuse this or any other symptoms with those of purely physical etiology, e.g., congenital lordosis. A working knowledge of medical conditions and surgical procedures with resulting physical disabilities is imperative. Occasionally patients have been referred for dance psychotherapy when the cause of their symptom(s) is physical in nature.

—tension: something or someone is on his back
—tension: fear of being ganged up upon or carrying on behind his back

Buttocks

—tension: fixation at the anal stage
— "tight ass": fear of losing inner parts of the body
— "tight ass": fear of anal castration
— "tight ass": latent or overt homosexuality
—tucked: like a dog with his tail between his legs, fear of aggression from behind

Legs and Feet

—symbolic of degree of support, balance, mobility, and thus an individual's sense of autonomy
—broad stance: defiance of authority
—broad stance: denial of insecurity
—legs closely pressed together: self-conscious, resistive to sexual impulses
—tonicity: often dependent on genital drives and conflicts
—feet placement represent individual's grasp of reality; e.g., light tenuous—on tiptoes, or clutching—toes digging into ground
—tension: conflict between guilt or fear and the desire to kick out
—dead feeling: doesn't feel like he can stand on his own two feet and be independent
—dead feeling: doesn't feel grounded, connected to reality

## GESTURES

There are countless examples of symbolic gestures which can be either interpreted universally or idiosyncratically. These processes depend on many factors; among them: (1) inherited predisposition, (2) sequences of experiences and the relationship placed upon them, (3) original fixational situation of a gesture, (4) original response made to a stimuli, and (5) the specific symbolic element in the situation,[5] (6) as well as the cultural disposition.[6]

G. W. Allport states that:

"Much behavior in the young child is sinkinetic; that is to say, his adaptive acts are accompanied by auxiliary movements. This seems to be a natural stage in the process of transition from adjustment with single limbs. In fact, Oseretzky finds these "Mitbewgengen" a serviceable index of inferior motor development. Sometimes, as Holt has shown, vestigial infantile movements persist throughout life and become motor idiosyncracies of the individ-

5. Maurice Korut, "A Preliminary Note on Some Muscular Responses of Diagnostic Value in the Study of Normal Subjects," *American Journal of Psychiatry*, II (1931–1932), p. 65.
6. *Ibid.*, p. 38.

ual. Many of these idiosyncracies of course, are quite specific and persist as 'symbolic gestures;' but they are at the same time further evidence that adult expression is not completely specialized or entirely free from early ties."[7]

## PHYSIOLOGIC ORGAN SYSTEMS AND PSYCHOSOMATIC DETERMINANTS

Psychiatric researcher in psychophysiology Felix Deutsch, M.D., relates that psychosomatic phenomena are universal. He proposes that "the human being is organized on the prototype of a single cell which also functions on the pleasure-pain principle. It follows then that when a state of displeasure occurs, it is managed by the individual's reactive phsyiological structure linked with the cessation of distress, so that, through repeated experiences of displeasure, cell modification ensues in which physiology becomes physiologic-psychology. "Whenever a cell responds physiologically, a response to a psychological stimulus is part of the total cell response. The opposite is also true."[8]

Thus symptomatic alterations can occur on a cellular level. These changes in physical functioning are pre-conscious and give symbolic expression to developmentally based repressed energy. The following represent examples of psychosomatically affected systems:

### Gastro-Intestinal[9]

Vomiting—oral resistance to incorporation
Ulcer—repression of oral receptive demands
Anorexia—oral phase fixation
Obesity—need for oral gratification; eating becomes sexualized, eating the "forbidden fruit;" fear of drive discharge, use of fatty tissue as protective armor
Constipation—anal phase fixation; retention of rage; feces become introjected objects
Diarrhea—anal compensation through generosity; readiness to sacrifice
Spastic colon—anal phase fixation; repressed aggresion

### Circulation

Circulatory alternations—anxiety; rage; sexual excitement
Chronic irritable heart—unconscious aggression and its fear; anger toward same-sex parent

7. Allport, *op. cit.*, p. 19

8. Felix Deutsch, M.D., *On the Mysterious Leap from the Mind to the Body.* (New York: International University Press, 1973) p. 132.

9. Material derived from Otto Fenichel, M.D., *The Psychoanalytic Theory of Neurosis.* (New York: W. W. Norton & Co., 1972) and is not considered inclusive of psyhosomatic dysfunction and possible interpretations.

Essential hypertension—increase instinctual tension; readiness for aggression
Migraine—frightened; readiness to accept blame; dependence on parents; sexual inhibition

### Respiration

Nervous coughing—discharge of repressed impulses; conflict regarding incorporation
Asthma—passive receptive longing for mother
Skin rash—frustrated longing that can't find discharge
Skin eruption—conflicts regarding exhibitionism
Psoriasis—sadistic impulses against self
Pruritus—sadistic impulses

### Urination

Enuresis—yearning for infant privileges
Cystitis—urethral sadistic fixation; urogenital repression of sexuality

### Sexuality

Hypersexuality—sexual excitement with inability to have orgasms
Don Juanism—dependency on narcissistic supplies
Vaginismus—fear of castration
Amenorrhea and dysmenorrhea—attempt at symbolic restitution of early losses

## THERAPEUTIC PROCESS

No symbolic investment of body parts, gestures, or internal psychosomatic dysfunction which the individual uses should go unnoticed or unutilized in the therapeutic process. These, when detected, can serve as invaluable data, particularly in determining the level of dysfunction. For example, a tightened buttocks: level of fixation 1½–2½ years; or a rhythmic gesture repetitively stroking an object, twirling hair, or fingering the mouth: level of fixation 0–1½ years.

Always ask the individual in question what the tension spot, gesture, pain, etc., means to him and what his associations are. All too often the person is overlooked and a highly idiosyncratic process is misinterpreted.

This dialogue cannot occur, however, until the symbolic process is brought into conscious awareness of the person. This may be carried out through experiences in sensory awareness, empathetic movement reflections by the therapist, suggestions for thematic movement improvisations which might amplify the symbolic content of the somatatization, personification of the organ or tense part and having it speak, or through pictoral representations of the area.

During the middle phase of therapy the individual explores the somatatization further in movement. Each time new facets and relationships to developmentally based patterns are delineated. The past is connected to present behavior and to the therapeutic relationship.

In the final phase, insight regarding the somatatization allows for the client/patient to disidentify from the behavior and explore through movement and other body-felt experiences, new, more developmentally appropriate ways of being-in-the-world.[10]

10. Bernstein, *Eight Theoretical Approaches in Dance-Movement Therapy. op. cit.*

# CHAPTER VI

# The Impact of Culture on Movement Behavior and Movement Therapy

The viewing of an individual's movement repertoire from solely a developmental-psychiatric standpoint without consideration of the cultural manifestations is a miopic and dangerous proposition (as dangerous as its reverse). All too often therapists look at motor behavior in terms of the presence or absence of pathology, the degree of physical and psychic integration, or the adaptability of the movement behavior without any thought as to the cultural implications. Compounding this is the fact that many of the above indicators are culturally biased—not to mention the effect of the therapist's own cultural patterns.

It is important that all clinicians take their heads out of the sand and view individuals and groups in a wider context. If these people are to work with an individual, an awareness of the values and resultant movement patterns that are culturally and economically significant for the patient are imperative. All too often, resocialization or therapy means the unsuccessful attempt of one group, one level of society, to channel another group into a stereotyped automaton of themselves.

People from different cultures and subcultures move differently. Weston La Barre in his study of the cultural basis of movement has proven that there is no "natural" universal language of shape flow design gesture and that it tends to be culturally determined.[1] Birdwhistle revalidates La Barre's results and further states that these movement patterns are "kinesthetic languages" which are learned by members of a culture as is the usual verbal method of communication.[2]

Alan Lomax, in conjunction with Irmgard Bartenieff and Forestine Paulay, compiled a study utilizing a cross-cultural analysis of movement parameters of fifty cultures.[3] From their many observations they were able to state: "The way that the present parameters sorted themselves out from a great

1. Weston La Barre, "The Cultural Basis for Emotions and Gestures," *Journal of Personality,* 16, 1947, p. 67.

2. Ray Birdwhistle, *Introduction to Kinesics,* (University of Louisville, Michigan, 1967), xerography, p. 65.

3. Alan Lomax, *Folk Song Style and Culture,* (Plimpton Press, Washington, 1968).

number of often most abstract subtleties during our research has convinced us that these descriptions of movement behavior actually extract the essential characteristics which differentiate different areas of humanity from another."[4]

The regions of culture-movement were reconfirmed by their folk song styles. Of more relevance, however, is the fact that, after studying the movement qualities of the "main activity patterns of everyday life and their function as a means of reinforcing and supporting the principal survival patterns of the culture," it was found that the movements required for the above manifested themselves in other areas of the culture such as play and particularly the dance style. This study has further shown that the main determinants of movement style variation seem to be the type of economy and the level of its complexity. Similarities of movements of individuals when not at work are drawn between various cultures which have the same types of subsistence economies.

Culturally determined social sanctions, government, degree of stratification, male-female interaction, and social relationships were also found to influence an individual's movement patterns. Movement, and dance specifically, serve as a training mechanism in the integration of various cultural elements. For example, anthropologist, Judith Hanna (1967) states, "African dances become meaningful and important in terms of their function as sources of cultural indoctrination, social control, and communication."

What does all this have to do with movement therapy? The jungles of Africa may seem far away from clinical settings. It is, however, quite relevant. This pure and relatively untouched dance style affords us an opportunity to view the use of movement without the complication of a "melting pot" society such as would be found in the United States or, for that matter, in a large part of the Western Hemisphere.

## MOVEMENT ANALYSIS OF CULTURAL PATTERNS

The study of African movement styles as a comparison will also allow us to trace the ancestry of Blacks who live in the U.S. Naturally there are differences within the total African profile; there are different subsistence economies, geography, etc. However, there are some easily traceable similarities which aid in the differentiation of European—American-European movement styles from that of Negro African and Afro-American.

One of the most differentiating elements is that of body attitude. The Black primarily uses his trunk as a two-unit system; Contrasting movement can be seen in the upper and lower halves of the trunk—whereas, the one-unit

4. Irmgard Bartenieff, "Research in Anthropology: A Study of Dance Styles in Primitive Cultures," *CORD, Research in Dance,* May 1967, p. 103.

system dominates the European (and Asian) population.[5] This factor alone can have a large effect on the diagnosis and treatment of individuals in these two continents.

Compounded with this is the discovery that Afro cultures generally utilize wider effort/shape variations than the European population. Blacks also rate higher in the use of flow[6] than do white European-Americans, demonstrating more spontaneity in their movement (Kestenberg).

W. C. Condon has filmed Whites, Blacks, and Black-White interactions to sort out, among other factors, the degree of movement synchrony between dyads. There appears to be more movement synchrony between White dyads and Black dyads with much less in Black-White communication. Condon also speaks of a "beautiful rhythmic pattern" between the Black dyads which, when this author observed, seemed to entail a large loading of synchronized flow attributes.

(It might also be important to note here that many Blacks have experienced much use of movement as a form of expression from early childhood, and may therefore feel more comfortable with its use.)

There are subtle European variations which also should be taken into consideration when working with different groups. Shape flow design is one of the major cultural indicators (Kestenberg). For example, there is a larger proportion of wide reversals into reach space (kinesphere) with Italians than with the French or English. There are differences within each country as well. The shape flow of the southern French, for example, seems to be a composite of northern French and Italian patterns.

To describe all the intricacies and tones of cultural and sub-cultural movement styles is not the purpose of this book or even this chapter. It would take a book in itself to come even close to this proposition. Rather, this author hopes only to draw the reader into a deeper awareness of and respect for the many parameters which are present.

Sorrowfully, very little work has been done in the study of the U.S.—most being done in the observation of more "pure" cultures. The United States is a cultural mixture, to be sure, and movement ethnographer-notators have shied away. The average American is a combination of many backgrounds and many environments. A good example of this is some of the white youth today who have incorporated characteristically Afro-American dance styles into their rock culture. Nevertheless, there are many patterns which remain and are transmitted via culturally biased parents to their children.

Anthropologist Benedict states in a study of child rearing practices: "Careful studies of mother-child relations have abundantly shown the infant's sensitivity to the mother's tenseness or permissiveness, her pleasure or disgust,

5. Lomax, *op. cit.*, p. 237.

6. *Ibid.*, p. 257.

whether these are expressed in her elbows, her tone of voice, or her facial expression. Communications of these sorts take place from birth on, and when a particular form of parental handling is standardized as 'good' and 'necessary' in any community, the infant has a greater multiplied opportunity to learn the traditional patterns."[7]

## NOTES ON MOVEMENT THERAPY APPLICATION

What does all of this mean for a dance-movement therapist? In general, it means he should take all of the above into consideration when diagnosing and establishing a treatment plan. Issues such as: is this individual going back to his subculture to live and/or work, or is he entering a new setting, one which requires a different movement style if communication is to be optimum. Discussion, films, and role playing with emphasis on non-verbal communication would be of help here.

Ideally groups should be divided culturally as well as in terms of adaptive pattern level.

The movement therapist should have a working knowledge of his or her cultural movement style and be able to adapt it when needed in order to afford greater synchrony and movement rapport with the client.

Music which is culturally familiar to the individual often has proven to be a comforting factor, particularly if he is in stange surroundings. Sharing a familiar song or melody with him can establish an avenue of communication which might otherwise not be open to the therapist. Culturally related music may also serve to draw him closer to his conflicts by triggering remembrances.

Use of the culture's stories, myths, and tales can be used to help assist individuals through their various developmental phases and life situations and can be enacted and explored for their cultural differences and universal application.

If there is one main idea from all of the above which should be remembered, it is this: No one cultural movement pattern is superior to another; movement which might be diagnosed as pathological in one country could be considered normal and even enviously desired in another (Paulay). Myopia can not only be a maladaption of eye functioning, but of perception as well.[8]

7. Ruth Benedict, "Child Rearing in Eastern European Countries," *Personalities and Cultures*. Robert Hunt, Ed. (New York: National History Press, 1967), p. 342.

8. Having no other related place to put this bit of information, but feeling it too important to discard, I am extracting Allport's list of "factors which may influence movement" as a gentle reminder and a prophilaxis against myopia: 1. Exigencies of immediate goal 2. Deformation of the body 3. Condition of health and disease 4. Individual peculiarities of muscular structure and body metabolism 5. Constitutional make-up 6. Age and sex 7. Strain and fatigue 8. Physical environmental conditions 9. Habits from special training 10. Racial tradition 11. Temporary social environment, leading to artificial manners or to a masking of normal expression.

## CHAPTER VII

# The Relationship of the Transpersonal to a Developmental Theory of Dance-Movement Therapy

The main thrust of developmental dance-movement therapy is the age-appropriate experience of wholeness. Many movement psychotherapies confine themselves to the intrapersonal-interpersonal dimensions of an individual's process of adaptive development. The roots of the theory of recapitulation of ontogeny stem from the ego psychologists, Eric Erikson, Heinz Hartmann, and Anna Freud, who stress ego reality as a primary focal point. There is, however, another point of view which shifts the focus from the ego as the sole mediating force and adds a third dimension to the dynamic matrix. This so-called third dimension deals with the relationship to those experiences which are beyond the individual and the space-force-time environment as is ordinarily experienced.

Movement psychotherapy which is influenced by the transpersonal recognizes the potential for experiencing a broad range of states of consciousness and adds to traditional areas and techniques "an interest in facilitating growth and awareness beyond traditionally recognized levels of health. In so doing . . . the validity of transpersonal experience and identity is affirmed."[1]

A three-dimensional model of dynamic movement psychotherapy can then be built, with the length being the intrapersonal process, its width being the interpersonal interface, and the depth/height being the transpersonal. See Figure VII.1.

The interpersonal dimension is viewed as a mirror for the individual's disowned unacceptable aspects of his psychology. Exploring through expressive movement themes the feelings of anger, love, fear, or disdain toward another, a group, an idea, or a phenomenon reflects projections from the unconscious. The interpersonal world explicates the influence of past, developmentally housed relationships with parents, siblings, and other significant figures.

1. Frances Vaughn and Roger Walsh, "Beyond the Ego: Toward Transpersonal Models of the Person and Psychology," *Synthesis*, Vol. 3–4, 1977.

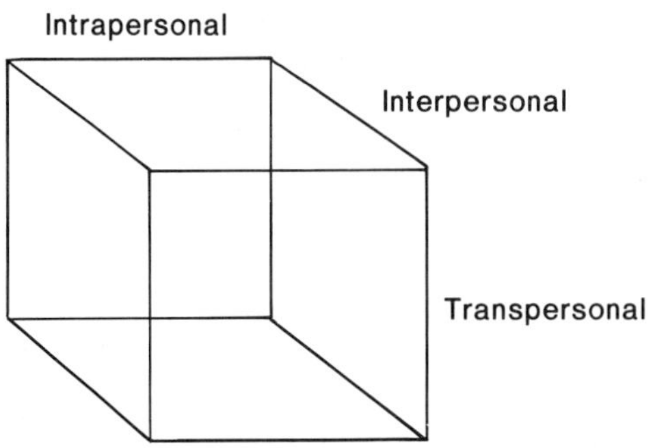


**Figure VII.1.**

The unintegrated parts of a person's intrapersonal dimension are manifested through the metaphoric language of primary process. It is through the arena of personal symbols and themes from movement active imagination experiences and other communications from the unconscious that developmentally related aspects of a person's psyche can be contacted.

The transpersonal dimension also utilizes the unconscious as well as the environment via synchronistic events as ways into an individual's experience.[2]

Universal instinctual material may emerge through a person's movement experiences manifested from the objective psyche. The acknowledgement of the existence of a so-called "objective" aspect of an individual's psychology goes beyond the view that an individual's unconscious is comprised solely of repressed drives and instincts. Contacts of a transpersonal nature transcend the individual's personal acquired understanding and allow access to fundamental information concerning humankind, the world, the universe, and the individual's relationship to them. A pool of universal cross-cultural archetypal symbols and mythologems are considered by Carl Jung to be part of the inherited structure of each person's collective unconscious.

These three dimensions then interrelate with one another as shown in Figure VII.2.

Each individual has his own unique way of experiencing this three-dimensional matrix. Some focus on one dimension to the exclusion of the others, but they eventually experience feelings of loss, emptiness, or poverty in the area(s) which has not been sufficiently integrated. The self-appointed guru who has inflated his ego by identification with the transpersonal wonders why he is incapable of personally relating to people. The spiritually impoverished business person who feels deeply that, in spite of his financial success,

2. Von Franz (1979) writes of such phenomena: "Where we normally live in a dual world of "outer" and "inner" events, in a synchronistic event this duality no longer exists: outer events behave as if they were a part of our psyche, so that everything is contained in the same wholeness." (p. 115)

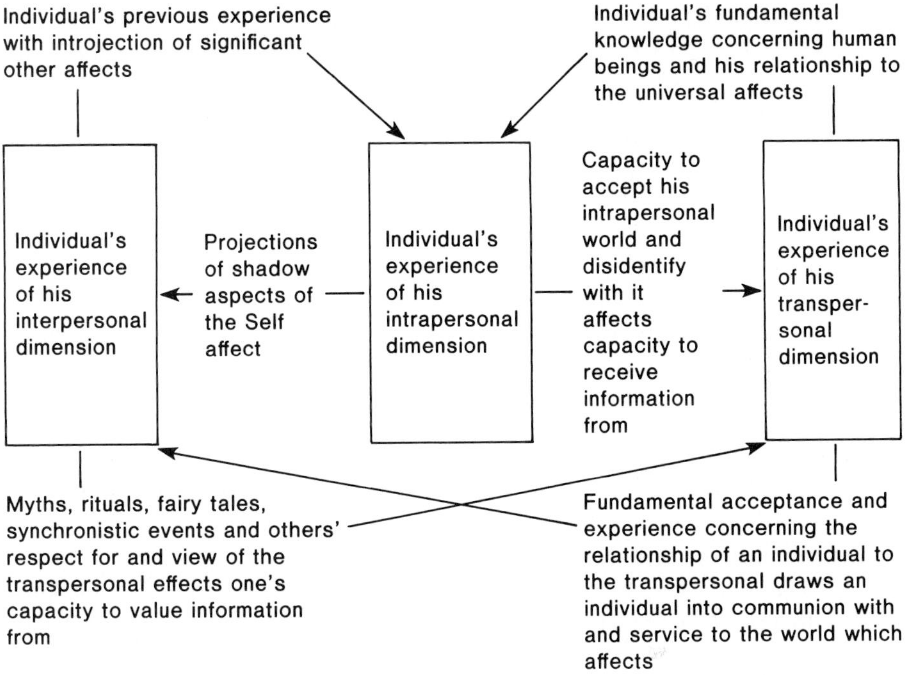


**Figure VII.2.**

there is something missing from his life. A ten-year five-day-a-week psychoanalytic veteran realizes that his decade of self-focus has not provided the total answer. These may all be examples of this state of imbalance. Other individuals work toward integration within these three areas simultaneously. The dynamic relationship among the three dimensions to the Self is represented in figure VII.3. This pyramidic structure is far stronger than two-dimensional support systems. The Self at the apex can only rest securely when all three sides have equal weight or value.

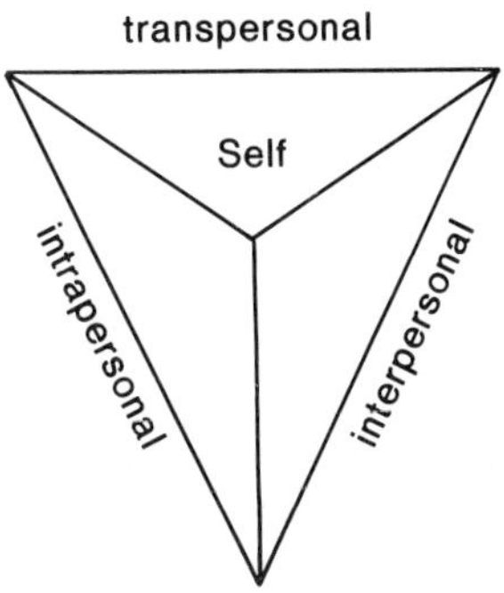


**Figure VII.3.**

History has demonstrated that in the earliest time a person would go to one individual to explore these three dimensions. The shaman was both priest and healer. In modern times, it is the work of Carl Jung which first provided a psychotherapy which accepted the "numinous dimensions of experience."

Jung continuously saw that, through synchronistic events and universal archetypal symbols and myths, there was a dynamic other than the intra- and interpersonal influencing the psychotherapeutic process. He writes:

"Archetypes have a distinctly numinous character which can only be described as 'spiritual' . . . it can be healing or destructive, but never indifferent."[3]

The central archetype is the Self. It symbolizes the totality of the personality in a state of consciousness.

The process of therapy or individuation can be greatly assisted by the Self. Through the Self, the individual is provided with a bridge between the psyche and the universe.[4]

The first stages in therapy often entail the disidentification of various aspects of the personality. Narcissistic personalities must recognize that they are not their personas; hostile male-hating women that they are not their animi; rational pragmatic businessmen that they are not their logical mediating ego. People *have* personas, animi/animae, and egos. "Disidentifying from the personality means recognizing experientially that our personality is not what we are, but what we have; not the source of our identity, but the means to express that identity in the world" (Ferman and Vargive, 1977, p. 76).

The persona, or mask an individual wears in order to be seen a certain way—the animus in woman representing her masculine side as well as her experience of men; the anima in man reflecting his feminine nature and his relationship with women; and the ego are all considered in Jungian psychology to be complexes. These and others like the father and mother complexes have central transpersonal archetypal cores of energy which are present at birth. As the child goes through the various developmental stages, phase-related relationships are cathected in the form of imageful psychic energy onto the associated complexes. Maladaptive behavior will cover and distort the individual's relationship to the complex. For example, if the personal mother was unable to nurture, to provide positive libidinal investment in the infant, and instead instilled rejection and guilt, the individual will often view the archetypal great mother as cold and inaccessible.

Part of the function of the therapeutic process entails the fostering of awareness, exploration, and the working-through of developmentally related

3. Carl Jung, *On the Nature of thePsyche* (New York: Bollingen Foundation, 1960), p. 115.
4. *Ibid.* p. 13.

maladaptive experiences so that the covering around the complex will be dissolved and the individual will have access to the archetypal core. In the case of the mother complex, the individual, through a non-directed movement improvisation, might have the experience of a presence of an all-loving, all-accepting womanly being who surrounds him with warmth and inspires a gentle, feminine inner-genital rocking rhythm in the individual's authentic movement.

Through this contact with the transpersonal dimension, intuitive hunches, archetypal dreams, synchronistic events, and perhaps visions or sartoris which do not have rational cause and effect or space time correlates will become accessible to the individual.

Energy from the transpersonal translated into these experiences serves several functions. On an intrapsychic level it often rattles the underpinnings of rigidified unintegrated pieces of the individual's psychology, shaking loose archaic orientations to the Self. It transforms the ego and other complexes and reorients them in relation to the objective psyche. Regarding the interpersonal dimension, Jung writes:

"There arises a consciousness which is no longer imprisoned in the petty over-sensitive, personal world of the ego, but participates freely in the wider world of objective interests. This widened consciousness is no longer that touchy egotistical bundle of personal wishes, fears, hopes, and ambitions . . . instead, it is a function of relationship to the world of objects, bringing the individual into absolute, binding, and indissoluble communion with the world at large."[5]

## RELATIONSHIP TO MOVEMENT THERAPY

It has been evident throughout recorded time that movement is one of the most primary vehicles for the experiencing of these three dimensions.[6] Intrapersonally, infants first learn about themselves through the movement of their bodies. Freud's statement that the ego is first and foremost a body ego directly relates to this process of experiencing oneself. Enactive cognition is the most fundamental manner of learning—far more basic than that of talking which entails abstract cognition, or even pictoral art which is on an iconic level of representation.

Secondly, movement, because of its primitive nature, can provide a direct avenue into the personal unconscious. Through body movement unconscious material can be expressed unedited by the ego.

Interpersonally, movement has been considered to be the most primary mode of communication. From the rocking of her infant by the nurturing

5. Jung, *op cit.*, p. 127.
6. Bernstein, *op cit.*, 1979.

mother to the kinesics of social interaction, body movement conveys the underlying, often more authentic messages of its bearer. Because of dance-movement's fundamental power as a vehicle for interpersonal relating, cultures have utlilized it in their communities' festivals, and dance therapists have employed it through empathetic movement reflection to relate with the most severely withdrawn and disturbed individuals.

Secondly, body-movement can tap into developmentally based, interpersonally related schemata and bring them into the foreground through metaphoric reenactment.

Transpersonally, dance-movement has been utilized in rites and rituals throughout the ages as a vehicle for transcendental archetypal experiences.[7] (The case study of Mark in Chapter IX is a prime example of this type of transformation.) "Every dance is a pantomime of metamorphosis which seeks to change the dancer into a god, a demon, or some other chosen form of existence. Its function is cosmogonic. The dance is the incarnation of eternal energy."[8] Through synchronistic rhythmic body action in group circle dance, individuals in countless cultures have been able to transcend the personal and mundane, affording participants contact with higher, more universal realsm.[9] Cirlot writes, "Dances performed by people with linked arms symbolize cosmic matrimony—the union of heaven and earth."[10]

## CASE STUDY

### Virginia

Groups are not a prerequisite for contacts with the archetypal. Virginia, a cultured active woman in her early forties who was engaged in short-term intensive movement therapy, can provide an example of the relationship of developmentally related material to the accessibility of reconnection with the transpersonal archetypal core. It was clear from her breathing, aligned body attitude, and rich movement repetoire that Virginia had already attained a high level of integration. However, a piece of her developmental history remained unintegrated.

Virginia's father, a charismatic powerful man, had divorced her mother and left the family system when she was engaged in the process of moving from puberty to adolescence. Developmentally the tasks associated with this

7. Ibid.

8. J. E. Cirlot, *A Dictionary of Symbols,* (New York: Philosophical Library, 1978).

9. Bernstein, *op cit.,* 1979.

10. Cirlot, *op cit.,* p. 77.

phase are not dissimilar to the initial oedipal period in which the child needs acknowledgement and positive acceptance of his or her emerging sexuality. In this second oedipal phase, the daughter often explores her burgeoning adult feminity with her father. He is the first man in her life, and his responses to her feminine development serve to reinforce and organize her genital sexuality. Overresponsiveness in the form of incestual advances or, as in the case of Virginia, an absence of the father or paternal significant other will cause maladaptive behavior to interfere with full intimacy and genitility.

Although Virginia had a successful marriage and had three children, she had an internal sense that a deeper integration could occur. She had been in classic Jungian analysis but felt it to be too "heady." She had brought in a dream which heralded her movement work and the psycho-physiologic transformations that would take place.

While moving during one of her initial sessions, she experienced an imageful kinesthetic sensation of having an extra, leather-like, outer layer of skin which covered her pelvic area and her thighs. She subsequently brought in a picture of herself encased in this leather. It had the look of chastity belts worn by the wives of the crusaders during the Middle Ages. She was aware that it was not static, that holes were developing in it allowing for the interpenetration of energy to occur. In another session the therapist suggested that she bring her father into the room. She spoke to him about her longing to be seen by him. She then grew silent, and a loosening of her bodily tension occurred. She described a feeling of experiencing an energy flow into her, and a sense of the entirety of her body emerged.

In a subsequent session she said she felt the need for roots. She had taken on the role of her father when he left the family and in doing so had over-developed her animus in relation to her feminine strength. Now she began a "root dance." Using gravitational weight efforts and flow, and with her pelvis and thighs initiating, she moved throughout the room. She looked like a fertility goddess fully engaged in a ritual process.

It was during the following session that contact with the transpersonal was made. The relationship to the personal father had been changed in such a way as to allow for an archetypal experience with the Father to ensue.

She began by sitting and moving slowly in the saggital dimension. Her torso was hollowed, her arms arched forward. Her movements became stilled and more subtle. There seemed to be an atmosphere of a numinous quality in the room. She later shared that she had experienced an indigo blue star-like energy coming into her head and moving down her torso. The color changed as it moved into her heart. It flowed slowly down to her coccyx and then exploded out and radiated through her entire body.

In a subsequent active imagination fantasy she floats in a circular pattern with a senex figure on top of a mountain. Soon this physical reality disappers and she is in the cosmos with one-celled "humanoid" life forms floating about her.

Virginia gradually began to value the subtle but deeply powerful movement experiences which emerged from her surrendering to her unconscious. During one of her last sessions she began by talking about how important it was for her to wait for the movement to emerge. She subsequently lay on her back with her legs bent and her feet on the floor. Her breathing seemed to initiate in her pelvis. After several minutes, she quietly moved to a kneeling position. Her arms first spread, then gradually enclosed in space. When at last she came back into the space, force, time reality of the room, she turned toward me. Her face radiated a soulful serenity. It was apparent that something both transpersonal and integrating had occurred. It would have been difficult not to be moved by her presence and the quality of energy that she was quietly allowing to flow into the room. Processing could wait. I made sure only that she was conscious enough to tackle the realities of driving her car and responding to the outside world.

During the next session she was able to relate what seemed readily apparent. She recalled a poem about the freedom of the feminine to choose her path and then said she had sensed an internal presence. She felt both awed and calmed by it. She spoke with a reverential quality in her voice. She had experienced the Self—the unifying force of the psyche which draws individuals into the transpersonal.

# CHAPTER VIII

# The Movement Therapist

Although the fundamental premises regarding the role of movement therapists are constant, their involvement in the process varies greatly depending on the population engaged in the therapy.

Basic to all work is the capacity to remain present and in synchrony with the client/patient(s). The therapist may have an acute sense regarding the path the individual needs to follow, but the person's own timing and direction decides the psychotherapy process. The therapist, however, is not limited to the sphere of secondary process reality. Often the best work is carried out when he allows his unconscious to merge with that of the client/patient. Empathetic intuition and the therapist's own associative fantasies are vital to enrich the process. This can only be undertaken if the therapist is able to allow his own ego boundaries to subside and to reform when the appropriate time comes for assisting the client in making conscious connection to his life.

## ROLE OF THERAPIST

Naturally, if a movement therapist has not sufficiently begun to recognize and accept a particular unintegrated constellation, he will have difficulty working with and encouraging related material from the client. If the patients primarily live in their own unconscious, as with psychotic individuals, they will readily know the world of the therapist's unconscious. It therefore behooves the clinician to be familiar with personal resistances, conflicts, and fixations. The deeper the therapist's experience, the deeper the client can explore. The therapist will have difficulty guiding individuals in their journeys if the paths and directions are unfamiliar territory. Personal depth therapy is an investment not only for the clinicians, but for their patients as well.

## CLIENTS

With individuals whose ego boundaries are functioning, the movement therapist's role is of an active receptive nature. These individuals, or clients as they will be called, are capable of forming a working alliance with the dance therapist. This relationship occurs with what Greenson calls the person's "reasonable ego." It is this part of the client's psychology that, no matter how deep the transference, is still able to rationally view the therapeutic process with perspective.

In order for the appropriate dyadic constellation or positive transference to develop, often a great deal of time needs to transpire. In therapy, a year is not an uncommon amount of time to wait before someone can begin to project his feelings toward past significant others on to the therapeutic relationship. Negative transferences emerging from the compulsion to repeat maladaptive parent-child phenomena can precede transferences which begin to positively organize and integrate developmentally related phases.

Classic psychoanalytic methodology categorically opposes so-called gratification of infantile needs. Although the approach presented here would argue that negative transferences are important developments in order for the individual to re-experience the significant unintegrated phase(s), providing the needed relationship for the person to begin to organize relevant developmental tasks might be considered by some to be in opposition to the psychoanalytic assumption.[1]

For example, in a positive oral mother or father transference, constructively reinforcing the person's body image or even touching or holding the client at specific points may provide the needed kinesthetic-sensate experiences to enable the person to construct a positive mother-child or father-child adaptive schema. Or during a positive anal transference, commenting on the movement "productions" of the client or reassuring positive regard during the client's self-assertions and aggressive expressions are part and parcel of the total therapeutic environment.

For the most part, however, creating space for the client's unconscious to explore the needed environment is the major role of the movement therapist. Interpretation of the symbolic material based on his related developmental tasks provides the bridge into the present use of adaptive patterns.

## PATIENTS

Those individuals who are unable to adapt to reality exist in the world of their unconscious. These persons are typically placed in institutional settings. The dance therapist's role with these patients, as they are called here, is often more physically interactive. The Chace approach employing movement empathetic reflection is often the style of choice. (See pages 13–14.) Through this approach an "alliance of unconsciouses" is formed. The dance therapist does not demand that the patient communicate in the clinician's

1. Greenson, Ralph, *The Technique and Practice of Psychoanalysis* (New York: International Universities Press), 1967.

language, i.e., secondary process verbalization, but rather stays with the method of communication in which the individual is engaged.

Here, both negative and positive transferences are enacted between the therapist and patient in dyadic movement adaptive activities. Since the psychotic individual already has access to his unconscious world, the role of the dance therapist is to continuously assist the patient in bridging the gap into his consciousness and in reclaiming his ego whose role it is to mediate inner experience with the outer environment.

## NOTES ON SUPERVISION

The role of dance therapist as supervisor of interns is not qualitatively dissimilar to that of clinician. Although it is important to insure that the relationship between supervisor and supervisee is not equated with that of therapist and client, the general orientation to the process can nontheless be viewed as analogus.

As with a client, it is vital to start where the intern is. Exploration of the intern's levels of expertise and anxiety, as well as of his fantasies and expectations regarding the internship, all need to be part of the horizon of the interactional phenomena. Establishing a contract among supervisor, intern, and facility allows for a clear commitment to the learning process. The style and methods of the supervision may need to be part of what is initially shared, just as a clinician's theoretical orientation may be relevant to the client's understanding of movement therapy.

This book has delineated a developmental frame of reference for working with clients and patients. Interns have their own developmental process from initial dependency upon the supervisor for role modeling to greater independence in which the supervisee interacts in the clinical setting in a relatively autonomous manner.

Typically there is a period of orientation in which the intern acquires a sense of the social system of the setting. Interns may participate in the therapist's sessions or view them through a two-way mirror. Co-leading may emerge with the gradual slackening off of the supervisor's role to that of participant/observer/consultant.

Actual supervision goes on formally on a regular weekly basis and typically informally as well. The intern is encouraged to develop his own style and theoretical frame of reference based on his psychology and movement repetoire. Generally, when suggestions are translated into questions which seek to draw the answers from the supervisee, responsibility for the emerging professionalism is maintained by the student while his mind is gaining experience in creative problem solving. In this way the supervisor, too, is afforded an opportunity to learn and experience new ideas.

## NOTES ON ADMINISTRATION

Administration is another one of those responsibilities which seem to creep into the realm of the duties of a movement therapist. "Successful administration is the creation of an environment which enables a group of qualified people to contribute toward a socially valued purpose to the fullest extent of their individual capacities and resulting personal satisfaction, growth, and fulfillment" (Group for Advancement of Psychiatry).[2]

In other words, effective administration facilitates the efficient and productive use of the staff and the facilities available. There are many ways of achieving good administration, but regardless of the vehicle, planning is one of the first steps. Definitions of who, what, where, how, and when, as well as policies, procedures, and methods, are usually better decided upon before a problem arises around them. Once these areas have been explored, some type of organization, no matter how small the department, must be established. Chains of command, specific job titles and descriptions, supervision, assignments, staff development, and equipment, layout, and supplies are all areas of attention. Once these have been worked through, the Dance Therapy Department is ready to carry out its function. The administrator, then, as coordinator and supervisor, facilitates avenues of communication and evaluates the effectiveness of the department.

### Personnel

Administrator—A DTR responsible for the "professional performance of the department's staff as well as the planning of overall treatment policies and procedures for patient treatment programs."[3]

Staff Therapist—full or part time, his first responsibility is the patient. He is responsible to the administrator and supervisor. Duties generally consist of patient care; collaboration with referring clinician, social worker, or any other staff related to the case; the writing of evaluations, treatment plans, and progress notes; and case presentations.

Supervisor—A DTR "directs and supervises staff therapists and other subordinate personnel,"[4] dance therapy interns, relates with graduate dance therapy programs, and provides on going written and verbal communication with these institutions.

Consultant—an individual who is highly qualified to give advice in a specialized field, e.g., dance therapy in the classroom as primary prevention, work with multiply-handicapped, trained movement analyst, etc.

2. Mosey, *Op. cit.*, p. 219.
3. *Manual on Administration* (New York: AOTA, 1965), p. 22.
4. *Ibid.*

Student Intern—the department is responsible for providing a student affilitation which meets the student's needs and the demands placed on him in his future work.

Aides, Orderlies, Attendants—in some institutions other staff members participate in the Dance Therapy experience. Communication with these individuals is imperative. Staff training and meetings scheduled to process groups in which they have participated may provide relevant avenues for understanding and learning.

### Physical Facilities and Equipment

*Space for:*

Offices

Storage of Equipment

Treatment Area—Many dance therapists choose to work on the floors where the patients live. Since the patients are most familiar with this area it often affords an atmosphere which is more conducive to therapy. In other situations, however, the reverse is true. Regardless, it is wise to have a room available for treatment. Even if the groups are led on the ward, individual treatment should take place in a separate room. Ideally the room should be large enough to accommodate the largest group without producing a "claustrophobic" reaction to moving in a cramped space, but not so big as to give a sense that there are no limits, no controls if needed. Acoustics, wood flooring or carpet (wall-to-wall so no one slips), and adjustable lighting is vital. One wall can have a full-length mirror which is large enough for at least two people to use, and there should be a curtain or panel to cover it when it is contra-indicated as an aid in treatment. A two-way mirror for observation is also a useful feature.

### Equipment

Record Player

Records—Basic records have traditionally been: waltzes; related folk (Hebrew, polkas, African, rock, Greek, Caribbean-Latin); music which doesn't superimpose its mood such as Indian, chants, or Impressionistic; mood music for anger, sadness, fearfulness, joy, tranquility, feeling big, small, light, heavy, slow, quick; and music to emphasize flow or full-effort actions such as flicks, dabs, glides, punches, slashes, floats, wrings, and presses. Special records which have particular meaning for individuals can also be invaluable. "White sound," chants, or mediation music is helpful when encouraging unconscious authentic movement. Music of a soothing, quieting nature is important to have, particularly at the end of sessions to calm individuals or to bring them back from unconscious movement experiences.

Percussion Instruments
Mats or Matresses
Pillows or Punching Bag
Stretch Rope or Stretch Circular Band
Towels
Parachute
Balance Board
Trampoline
Balls
Two-color materials such as ribbon (left-right discrimination)

Two-color tile squares to place on the floor (foot placement with left-right discrimination)

Various modular forms (for making obstacle course, imaginary scene, or stage)

Various texture of floor tiles (texture discrimination)
Hula Hoops
Weights (type that wrap around wrist and ankles)

Various objects for duplication of movement qualities such as scarfs, balloons, rock, aluminum foil, rubber, clay, etc.

Various fabrics, masks, hats, and costumes etc., for dramas in movement.

Regardless of the patient's age, a pool is a marvelous facility to have available. If there is one existing at or near the facility, be sure to section off some time for its use.

### Clothes

Clothes, like the way one stands and moves, send off non-verbal messages to individuals in the environment; so it is important to be sure of what you want to say! Also, constant variation in clothing can sometimes have an adverse effect on patients. To some of them, the environment is at best confusing. A familiar person in familiar clothing is a comforting relief.[5]

### Interdepartmental Administration

The coordination of all the departments for the proper functioning of the institution is the major goal of interdepartmental administration. One tool which facilitates this is communication. However major difficulties frequently arise in this area. Much communication between departments is ritualistic.[6]

5. Autistic children are particularly sensitive to any change in their environment and that includes a change in the therapist's clothes.

6. Mosey, *Ibid.*

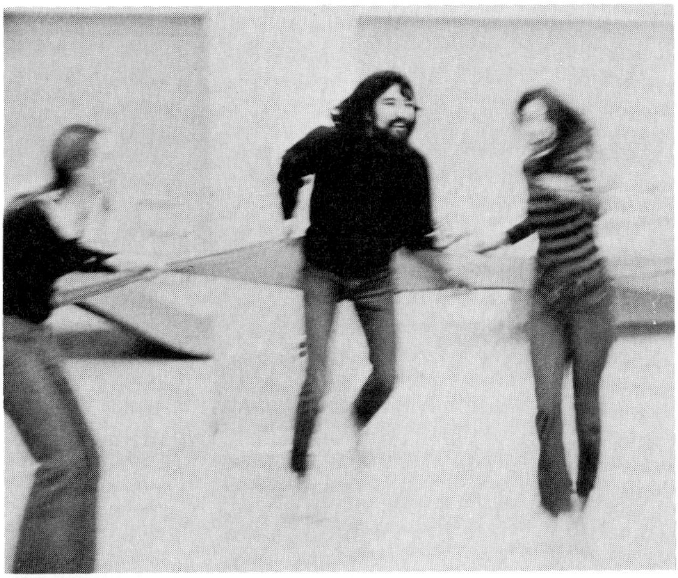

Stretch band

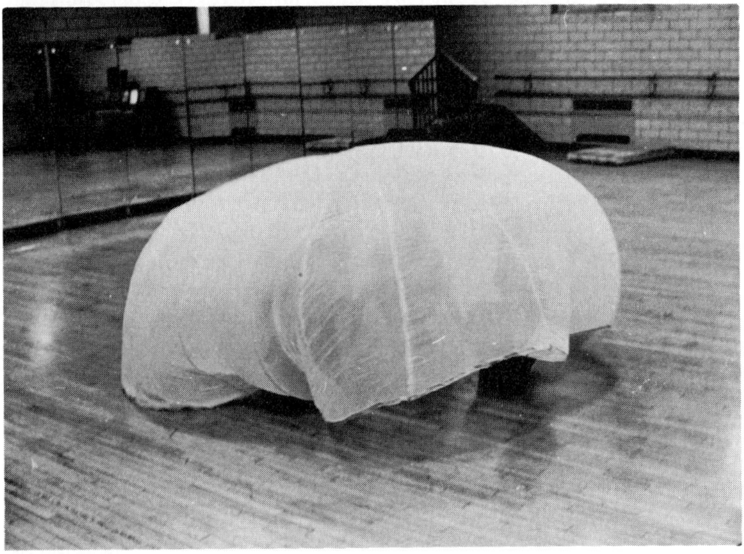

Parachute

Figure VIII.1.

More often than not, professionals accommodate each others' differences and show little concern or interest. Power struggles develop, and those who are not comfortable with themselves and their clinical roles often feel threatened by others, particularly if it seems the "others" are more successful than they. Physicians are no exception to this either; and if a doctor feels threatened by the movement therapist, the therapist is confronted with a problem.

There are many ways to handle this particular situation—one of which is not to handle it at all, which, of course, will be discarded immediately! Growth in interdepartmental knowledge of Dance Therapy, as well as of one's status and that of the profession, can be easily stifled by blocking this issue. If another movement therapist replaced him, he or she would have to work twice as hard to move himself out of this "defunct" position.

One way to deal with this problem is for the dance therapist to admit that he doesn't know everything and that he doesn't look to another therapist—be he doctor, psychologist, etc.—for omniscient panaceas and solutions to all problems. Once the therapist senses the dance therapist's sharing, non-threatening, relaxed manner, he may realize that he is not expected to be "SUPERTHERAPIST" and can begin to transfer some of the energy he employs for this defense to more productive use. Perhaps, also, if a dance therapist could come to terms with some of his own anxieties (if he has any, that is), this process of communication would be much easier. In movement terms, if flow is added to his repertoire, whatever it is, a person is at least halfway there.

# CHAPTER IX

# Case Studies

### Betsy

Betsy was a 17-year-old institutionalized adolescent diagnosed as having an adolescent depressive reaction. She was referred to the movement therapist by a psychiatrist who continued seeing her in therapy. It was decided that Betsy would be seen individually once a week by each therapist.

Initial observation-evaluation in an interactional session showed Betsy to have a great deal of maladaptive behavior in the flow of breath area. Her breathing was shallow and held at times of stress. A high degree of tension was present in the jaw and mouth. Her verbalizations were tight and whispered. She seemed to alternate between a sad smile and a sustained biting of her lips.

She was able to move utilizing the various effort/shape elements; however, there was no presence of posture-gesture or gesture-posture mergers in flow or effort/shape. Puppet-like behavior with tense artificial movements replaced P–G flow in situations where the merger would cathect psychic somatized material with which she was not ready to bring into conscious awareness. It was clear that many of her movement patterns were of an anal sadistic nature, particularly in the peri-oral region, making it even more difficult for her to yell out. Her negative body-image was reinforced by the intense retroflexed rage she kept within herself. In terms of drive-object organization, her fear of letting go was also shown in her subtle passive-aggressive behavior. Cognitive representation and perceptual areas of function were all intact. The dyadic relationship commenced on a semi-autonomous level.

Betsy's self-portrait (which was also used for diagnostic purposes) showed an unhappy face scantily attached to a wavy asexual body. The phrase "she didn't have a leg to stand on" clearly applied.

#### Rx: Immediate Goals

1. Increase flow of breath
2. Posture-gesture flow
3. Positive affect investment with emphasis on the release and integrated awareness of retroflexed rage (Body-image, Drive-object)

### Long-Range Goals

1. Sexual identity stage (Body-image).
2. Increase tolerance for inner genital rhythms with eventual genital rhythm integration (Flow Rhythm).
3. Appropriate investment of aggressive drives (Drive-object)
4. Autonomous relationship (Dyadic)
5. Merging of P-G and G-P effort/shape (Effort, Shape, Posture-Gesture)

The sessions often began with interactional movement patterns evolving into use of a strong, quick, direct pattern. Trust developed when Betsy was allowed to work through her pent-up anger in psycho-motor situations in which the therapist would cower in defeat as the aggressive object while being "destroyed" with punches, kicks, slashes, and angry verbiage. It was after these situations that Betsy was able to verbalize most freely, viewing with more realism her relationship with the individual(s) in question.

Shortly after starting, Betsy began bringing in favorite records which were charged with associations for her. Many sessions were started by both her and the therapist singing and moving to Carol King's "You've Got a Friend." The singing and dancing in synchrony reiterated the content of the song and further reinforced the contract. After a while Betsy also brought in dreams which were explored in movement and verbally processed. The gestalt hypotheses of dreams was utilized, i.e., that every aspect (object, person, etc.) of a dream is part of the individual himself. Through personifying various elements in her body attitude and movement, she was able to move clearly, understand the heretofore bound internal conflicts, separate the issues and emotions, and resolve them.

As she grew to feel more positively about herself, she was able to evolve a chumship level of relating to the therapist. Discussion of hair styles, clothing, and ways of relating to the opposite sex enhanced her emerging sexual identity, as did such suggestions as, "How would someone dance if she didn't want to be appealing . . . " now, "How would she dance if she *did* want to be appealing?" It was during experiencing the latter that Betsy, for the first time, willingly looked in the mirror at herself with a smile, while moving in an adaptive effort-shape gesture-posture merger to a favorite rock piece.

## Jim

Jim was a five-year-old diagnosed as having an adjustment reaction. He was seen solely by the movement therapist in individual sessions in a children's day treatment center. Jim's initial evaluation was through a two-way mirror, giving the therapist an opportunity to notate using an adapted Kestenberg Movement Profile.[1]

### Pre-effort/Directional Shape

Jim was continually acting suddenly, but showed very little intensity in his actions. Gentleness was the primary pre-effort utilized and was coupled frequently with suddenness. Little or no pre-effort investment was placed in exploring or communicating; he would seem to act before examining or clarifying his feelings. When the pre-effort graph was compared with that of the directional shape, the obvious dissimilarity between the corresponding elements denoted that he reacted like a "shot gun" with no intention as to where his movement was to be directed. Directional shape was primarily in the vertical. Although he seemed to exhibit a good deal of downward movement, there was little or no correspondence in pre-effort dynamic attached to it. He seemed to have his "head in the clouds" rather than his "feet on the ground." The load factors (complexity and sophistication of each movement) were 38% in pre-effort and 45% in directional shape, indicating a child of average intelligence.

### Rhythms

When the effort-shape graphs were compared to those of flow rhythms, affinities (oral-spacial effort, horizontal shape; anal-weight effort, vertical shape; urethral-temporal effort, sagittal shape) appear to be lopsided as well. There was a heavy loading of oral, oral sadistic, and inner genital libidinal rhythms, suggesting that Jim was still struggling with early maternal dependency. Aggressive behavior was thus expressed only at the oral level. He seemed to have acquired vertical movements via his identification with his mother rather than from related anal rhythms. This fixation was further born out by the fact that 6 out of 7 mixed rhythms have either oral, feminine, or both components. The sequential patterns of his rhythms showed Jim gradually working himself up to more outer genital rhythms proceeded immediately by more inner genital rhythms.

### Summary

The adapted profile showed a dependent 5-year-old who continually acted in a darting sudden manner without investment or forethought, which denoted a desire for, but fear of, aggressive behavior, as well as a possible counterphobic reaction of rushing into danger.

1. See "Outline for Movement Profile" in Appendix.

Rx

1. Increase verbal awareness of motor behavior (Thought process)
2. Outer genital rhythm (Flow rhythm)
3. Purification of rhythms (Flow rhythm)
4. Increase attention span (Effort/shape)
5. Broaden pre-effort profile particularly: gentle-sudden to vehemence-sudden and gentle-hesitation
6. Investment of aggressive drive in external objects (Drive-object)
7. Semi-autonomous relationship with therapist (with the placement of demands on the appropriateness of behavior) (Dyadic)

Treatment commenced with the formulation of an egocentric relationship with the therapist. The therapy sessions, for the most part, took the form of movement-drama interactions. Imaginary symbolic situations were utilized to work through more age-appropriate expression of feelings as well as to readapt a lopsided profile. The primary image chosen by Jim was that of a monster. The therapist was at first the object of the monster's oral aggressive behavior, but after a short period of time, the therapist was asked to become a "fellow monster" and "good mother" working with him to resolve some of his oedipal fears, so that he was finally able to identify with a more masculine age-appropriate repertoire. During this process he was weaned away from mother monster from his oral sadistic expression of anger, to that of the utilization of outer genital rhythms and more intensity in his dynamics. Initially, after Jim's battles with the male monster, he would curl up in a lair that he and the therapist would construct. There, sucking serenely on a baby bottle, he would be rocked by the mother-monster-therapist. Later, as the elements needed for the Oedipal situation to be resolved were explored and re-explored, Jim began to identify the therapist as a male-pal and co-construction worker. Large, real and fantisized edifices were built, torn down, and reconstructed. He was beginning to relate to the therapist as chum and to explore what Erikson terms successful industry. (See Appendix for delineation of Erikson's stages.)

As the therapeutic process continued, he could maintain his attention on one fantasy for the full one-hour session. There were periods of quiet with more deliberate movements as well as further needed clarification of rhythms.

Demands had also been placed on Jim in the way of suggestions for variations in his movement patterns, e.g., "Let's creep up on him (policeman, doctor, male monster) very slowly so he doesn't hear us, and then pounce on him with all our might."[2] Jim's verbilization increased from one- and two-

2. These male figures were father substitutes for Jim and were used to resolve his oedipal strivings.

word responses to elaborate descriptions of fantasies. Much of the verbal integrative process was conducted via the therapist talking to an imaginary figure, explaining to the figure why Jim could be mad and how in various situations he had a right to his feelings.

## Mrs. G.

Mrs. G. was a 72-year-old widow who was referred to the movement therapist for treatment in a geriatric psychiatric facility. She was seen individually by a psychotherapist as well as in a group in which the movement therapist was co-leader. Mrs. G. was diagnosed as having a depressive reaction and as being in the beginning stages of senility. It was decided that she be placed in a group after an initial period of individual sessions.

Mrs. G. was seen by the therapist in an evaluation session. Her fear regarding the loss of her memory was prominent. Every few minutes she asked where she was and if someone knew where to pick her up. Her movements were stiff and tense, similar to a wooden soldier's. She was extremely fearful of falling, which made her even more prone to do so. It was as if she had renounced the free flow of tension when using any of the complete effort-shape combinations. Even at the gestural level she was unable to experience these dynamics without tensing and going into bound flow.

Rx

1. Restore her movement repertoire (E/S, P-G)
2. Increase flow and relaxation (Flow of breath)
3. Provide for expression of feelings of fear and anger (Drive-object)
4. Egocentric group

Mrs. G. seemed to improve daily. An initial repetitive dance dyadic interaction was maintained by the therapist to reinforce her memory of the experience. The one-to-one also afforded the opportunity to center on the release of some of her feelings. Gradually she remembered and would look forward to the Dance Therapy sessions with great joy. As she entered the group experience, she began to encourage the other group members. As tensions were released from her body, her movement repertoire began to manifest itself again. She would lead the group into quick patterns changing into jumps and hops. Her fear of falling had disappeared and was replaced by an agility which was uncanny for a woman of her age and size.

(Mrs. G. was assigned to a mixed group of individuals with similar backgrounds, ages, and problems. Music which related to her youth was played to bring back and reinforce her previous movement repertoire as well as to cathect associations which would facilitate verbalization.)

## Movement Therapist as Movement Assessment Consultant

*Family Movement Evaluation*

| | |
|---|---|
| Family worker | |
| mother | father |
| identified patient | movement therapist |

Normally an evaluation of this sort is carried out by viewing a videotape or film which shows all the individuals involved fully at all times. If this is impossible, the therapist-notator generally observes interaction from behind a two-way mirror. Both of these alternatives were impossible in this setting, so minimal notational data was collected. This evaluation has been included to demonstrate how much an observer can pick up from a 30-minute session.

(The client is a 25-year-old male, diagnosed as a possible borderline personality. The above chart represents the family seating arrangement.)

Fred's (patient) body was characteristically in a bound rigid state. He exhibited only peripheral gestures in the forearms and legs; however these movements were, for the most part, devoid of dynamics. His seated posture was hollowed and shortened. His general shaping seemed to correspond to that of his mother's. She, in turn, was giving negative non-verbal cues to Fred which were watched carefully by him. For example, when asked by the family worker how she felt about Fred, she hollowed and shortened her abdomen stroking it as if she were in pain. Fred acknowledged his mother's non-verbalizations by moving his leg toward her when she spoke. It was difficult to determine by his ambiguous position whether he was blocking her or taking her in. Initially, Fred did not respond to his father at all (who attempted to take on his son's posturing, but, in contrast to the son's even flow, moved constantly in urethral rhythms). However, after about 20 minutes (in which the father constantly verbalized positive responses concerning Fred), Fred began to take on the same rhythm pattern in the calf of his leg which was closest to his father, as well as to move it toward his father when he spoke.

### Summary

Fred exhibited an immobilized torso throughout. No verbalization was made by him; his breath was shallow. When asked a question by the group worker, he would go into a high-intensity bound state. No flow adjustments were made except on a peripheral level. He seemed to be an extremely controlled, angry, fearful young man struggling with dependency needs toward his mother and an emerging identification with his father.

## Group Study

Since the group that will be discussed is not a typical Dance-Movement Therapy group, it is necessary to briefly outline what is felt to be a "classic Chace format" for the dance therapist. The following is what has generally been utilized with hospitalized patients. Although effort-shape terminology has been used, this format is also followed by those therapists who do not employ these concepts to describe their sessions.

Classic Dance-Movement groups generally involve an initial warm-up period in which the therapist, having gotten everyone together in a circle, commences the session by leading the group into a flow pattern (movements with no dynamics or spacial attributes). The goals are (1) to relax the group, and to "start the flow going," i.e., circulation with attention drawn to the body; (2) to provide a common movement pattern for all—one which is primary and can be observed in even the most regressed individuals; and (3) to provide a "blank canvas" upon which the patients might begin painting an expression of themselves. If the group consists of severely disturbed individuals, the flow can be initiated distally (hands and/or feet) and gradually evolved to include the whole body (a more postural pattern).

The therapist then looks around the circle and starts picking up and reflecting dynamics and shape which the patients or clients start to superimpose. If, for example, an individual starts to use quickness and indirectness along with flow, the therapist will empathetically attune to the pattern communicating to that member that she is with him. At this point the second phase of the therapy session begins.

The goals of the second phase are (1) to pick up and enlarge upon patterns which manifest themselves in the patient's repertoire toward (a) externalized drives and (b) more postural merger; (2) to attempt to include experience in all possible effort-shape combinations; and (3), given the above two goals, to bring the group to various emotionally expressive peak experiences followed by an evolution into more neutral, less charged movements.

Thus the therapist might evolve the above mentioned pattern of quickness and indirectness into use of a weight factor (strength or lightness). If none appears in the group, the therapist might choose the more indulging of the two as in this case it is the initial full effort pattern to be introduced. Thus a flick is utilized (quick, indirect, light). From this, if there is no observed change into an alternate dynamic by individual(s) in the group, the therapist might gradually change the intention toward space to produce a dab (quick, *direct,* light), and then if possible into a punch (quick, direct, *strong*). Shaping is dealt with concomitantly, as is experience with more postural and gestural patterns.

After a period of time experiencing this full fighting effort, the therapist will look to see if anyone in the group is changing any of the dynamics, shape, or body involvement. If so, he might then pick up on that pattern and evolve the group into another experience.

Within this second phase, dyadic or small group interaction sometimes occurs, depending on the level of the group. The circle may come together, spread apart, move into a line like a train moving about the room, or break up and come back together. Imagery and verbalization is encouraged to further assist in personal connection and expression. Themes are picked up and explored from the associations of the members of the group. Improvisations are suggested and geared to the level of the group's functioning.

The third phase often involves a period of diminishing work with the goals of (1) insuring return of individual control mechanisms.[3] and (2) drawing the individual into inner awareness of what has occurred in terms of perceptual feedback body awareness, cognitive realization, and integration of the emotional expression. This is often carried out via a rest period in which music of a more relaxing pensive nature is played. It has also been brought about via a toning down of the movement into a whisper—one which is brought about by use of more indulging efforts (light, slow, indirect) with gradual evolution into flow. Group hugs are not infrequent in a group of long standing followed by verbal sharing and exploring the relationship of imageful movement expressions and themes to their past and present lives.

## Analysis of Group

The group that will be discussed here consists not of hospitalized individuals, but rather of students and fellow mental health workers who were interested in learning more about themselves and dealing with conflict areas through the use of Dance-Movement Therapy.

The first portion of the initial session was devoted to establishing the contract for the weekly 3½ to 4 hour group. Self-awareness, conflict processing and resolution, the development of a more adequate body-image and more adaptive movement repertoire, as well as experience in interacting and being aware of others on a non-verbal level, were brought up. During this discussion it was established that each member would maintain his own responsibility for letting known his desire, to explore a certain area, and, if the group agreed, to then work toward bringing the behavior or unconscious material into figure. This was as simple as changing a record or as complex as wanting to work on

3. Often wards prefer the patients to be less expressive, feeling that expressive behavior interrupts the daily regime.

a problem area with the assistance of the group. The amount and form of the fee was also a personal decision.

The dance-movement therapist's role was clearly stated. She was to be a facilitator—one who would respond to the needs of the group by suggesting ways to explore and work through a particular need or problem area. She stressed the individual maintenance of responsibility for letting their needs to be known as well as for joining in or not in various processes in which other group members were interested. If the group or individual asked to deal with a certain area and if that area required a more structural approach, then, if all agreed, it would be used. However, no structure would be imposed unless asked for by group members.

Agreements were also made that, barring physical injury, destruction, and others trying to take over another's responsibility as to what or how he "should" work, the "door was open." An implicit contract was also made that individual crises took priority over what was occurring at that moment.

The group then opted into moving. A record was chosen by one of the members, and each person was given a self-decided period of time to move in his own way while others followed, sharing the person's feeling with him—each taking time to be with and getting to know each other.

The initial subsequent sessions were all structureless. These entailed the individual's entering the wooden floored, mirrored room and essentially waiting, getting in touch with his body and his wants, till he felt like moving. One or two members might choose a record and start dancing. Another might join with them while another might wish to be on his own. Still another might stay seated for awhile near the door sensing his own timing for involvement. For some, it was a new experience to gradually become aware of where, what, when, how, and with whom they *really* did want to move. Without pressure or demands, people began moving in ways they had either forgotten or had never experienced before.

As the group became more comfortable with their own movement needs and experimentation, individuals who had been "loners" started interacting with others in dyads and small groups. Sessions were followed by a period of discussion in which sharing and feedback occurred.

During this period the therapist's role was that of a supporter. She spent time moving with each individual, dancing with them in synchrony, letting them know that she could be with them, that they could be together. With some, the communication would evolve into reciprocal diagonal jabs at each other or mutual shoulder pushing. At other times communication would take the form of a rocking pattern while maintaining eye contact for minutes at a time.

When individuals seemed to want a group experience, e.g., triads drawing together, the therapist attempted to gently draw others who seemed willing into the interaction. This sometimes meant widening the circle, holding out an arm, incorporating someone into the elastic stretch rope, or gradually evolving an individual into the movement pattern of the group.

The therapist's role also consisted of being aware of when it was beneficial to "be" with a member and when it was important to allow someone to be by himself during periods of discovery.

Although the members of the group had well functioning control mechanisms and ego systems, the eye "in the back of the therapist's head" was always open. On occasion, experience in novel situations—situations in which there has been minimal experience in the utilization of controls—can produce new and sometimes frightening sensations in an individual.

After this initial foundation of familiarity and trust had been established, the group began to ask for structure which would further facilitate growth. Concurrently, individuals and dyads began verbally asking the group if they could "work." At these times, the therapist suggested various techniques to be utilized depending on the needs and problems. Gestalt, neo-Reichian, Jungian, and psychodramatic movement therapy methods were often used. Situations were restaged using members of the group. Other members observed these processes and identified with the various roles. On another occasion part of the group pinned an individual to the floor to help him to externalize the negative aspect of a conflict area and to personify more adaptive modes of behavior in a motorized exaggerated working out of being buried. At other times the whole group became involved in doing a certain exercise of which an individual was in particular need.

In this phase, the therapist's role was more directive, but she always reminded the individuals that she could not "make something happen;" She could only suggest a way and guide them through the process, and the rest was up to them. She also stressed the importance of their sensing their own "right time" to move, keeping watch that the group's incentive did not override the individual's. Her role was also that of caretaker, making sure that no one left the sessions in a disorganized or defenseless state. Each member knew that the therapist would be there to talk and/or work with him until he felt comfortable enough to depart.[4]

Thus if the reader recalls the Primary Group Levels of Organization, he will find this group progressing from a one-to-one parallel level, to a task

4. When the set time is over in many groups (or individual sessions for that matter), many therapists will usher their client(s) out the door, even if the individual is in the middle of a process. This is considered acceptable procedure of many. My own personal feeling is that the imposition of such a time superstructure often detracts from the therapeutic process as well as the relationship. The contact of "I will listen or be with you for one hour, but at the end of that time my ear and self is dead to you till next week," is in my opinion, bizarre when the person is essentially being asked to respond and interact in a "spontaneous" manner.—P.B.

level, to that of an egocentric group cooperative level in which members attend to each other's needs and respond by taking on various roles to facilitate another's working through of an area of concern.

### Helen
### Battle for Spring: An Initial Session

I have often been asked by my students "How do you begin with a client? What do you do? What do you say?" These questions seem to be of particular importance when in private practice where the referral to Dance-Movement Therapy may be as general as, "I think this individual could benefit from work with you." Here there is usually no chart, no nurses to consult, and no access prior to the session to observe and possibly notate the individual's movement sequences to ascertain a profile.

Such was the case with Helen who phoned one afternoon to make an appointment. With adequately functioning adults, people who seek help because, as Bernstein puts it, "You don't have to be sick to want to feel better," I feel in many instances that I have an ally against dysfunction. We exist within a partnership and share in the responsibility for the goals and the process of working toward them. Therefore, my "colleague" and I crystallize the maladapture behavior, evolve the contract, and select the method of therapeutic adaptive activities together. Utilizing strong eclectism in approaches under one frame of reference avails the client several alternative routes to awareness and function.

#### Initial Therapy Session:

We sat together for the first portion of the session and I asked her what brought her here, and what she felt she would like to work on. Helen, an overweight, sluggish woman in her 40's, shared with me, "My back has been aching and I've realized that putting on BenGay is not going to help.',

I suggested that the sustained removal of her backache be at least an initial goal in therapy and that we could work from there. She agreed. I then suggested several ways to work, thus affording her part of the responsibility of selecting the technique. Movement improvisation, classic Gestalt, breath release neo-Reichian patterns, body correctives, and massage were the avenues offered. She selected one of the more passive methods, massage.

Helen lay on her stomach and I began massaging her back, pressing and releasing with the flow of her breath. The painful area was easily found both visually and by touch. The muscles of her scapula girdle were bound and cold to the touch. Her breathing was excluded from this area as well.

"If your upper back pain could talk, what would it say, Helen?", I asked. She replied, "I keep her down . . . keep her from experiencing spring

. . . from being happy and from getting in touch with her own strength." She then made an allusion to a part of Solomon's "The Song of Songs" in the Bible, a metaphor to spring, "The season of glad songs has come, the cooing of the turtledove is heard in our land."

I noticed that her feet were becoming more bound as she tensely intertwined them with wrings (strong, sustained, indirect movement). I touched them; they were extremely cold from the lack of circulation.

As I rubbed them, she spoke, "I am Helen's feet. I'm afraid. I'm afraid. I tense up every time she tries to stand on me. My toes curl up. I won't let her stand on her own two feet. She'll have to depend on other support."

I suggested that she stand; and as she did, the tension rose up her legs.

"Walk around and allow whatever feeling with its voice to evolve." Her step became stronger, quicker, and more direct. I encouraged her to stamp; and as she did the voice of her foot tension could be heard, "I won't budge! I won't budge!"

I noticed that her arms lacked the strength of operation. Her shoulders were cutting off their power, producing a flailing pattern. Moving with her in synchrony, I assisted her into a posture-gesture merger of the flow of her breath coordinate and initiate the movement from the center of weight.

Helen was still internally conflicted; part of her wanted to move, to stand on her own two feet and to be independent, while the other part wanted her to remain dependent and helpless within the gestalt. I attempted to externalize the defense by becoming the part of her that wanted her to remain blocked.

"Don't move! You won't move!" I yelled in a P-G merging pattern. "I will move!" she retorted in a similar pattern. We continued till it seemed Helen had felt this side of her assert itself throughout her whole body.

After having her stand in a now more centered stance sensing the vibrations of her re-claimed body, she relaxed supine on a foam mat. From this position the throbbing of her jaw and neck could easily be seen. Both utilized an extreme bound flow in order to block her feelings from conscious recognition and expression. Helen still felt the conflict battling in her jaw: a desire to express aggression orally (perhaps in its primitive form to bite out and snap at someone), with a counteracting attempt to hold that expression back.

I suggested the bio-energetic technique of biting and holding a towel with her teeth and jaw. This seemed to protract and release some of the tension such that I felt she could begin to express and release this localized, repressed affect. We began moving in synchrony on all fours, glaring and snapping at each other like lionesses. She was encouraged to breathe deep into her pelvic girdle and allows growls to emerge.

As the activity seemed to come to a natural termination I suggested to Helen that she find a place in the room and a body position that seemed comfortable to her and to then allow herself to draw her attention inward. I asked her to move her awareness throughout her body and to seek out part or parts which she felt less than others, which may be numb, colder, more tense, or tingle. These areas are often "cloudier" in terms of readily available visual fantasies. However, I asked her to see if any images came to mind when centering on the identified areas.

After several minutes, Helen shared with me that she had an image of a tight umbilical cord wrapped around her cervix. She said that she was keeping her children tied to her with this cord, as well as having it tie off her unreleased anger and sadness at being unable to allow herself to experience her own spring—her re-birth.

I said that she looked sad, and slowly, tears began to appear. After a while I mentioned that sadness often comes from feelings of loss. She then spoke of the process of losing her old identity and of evolving toward a new one. It seemed to me that there were two conflicted parts in Helen, one which wanted to keep her in a static identity, in "winter" as she symbolized it with all the cold anger, sadness, and fear locked inside—the part that keeps her umbilical cord and bound tension in her body; and the other part which seems to be getting tired of the pain—the part that brought her to seek help—the part that wants her to grow, to be re-born.

I suggested that perhaps the contract could be expanded to include the resolution of these two aspects within the gestalt so that her body would not have to continue to be a battleground for the assaults and counter-attacks of these polarities.

In a sense, this was Helen's fight for her "spring"—for her Easter, as she put it. "It has been 42 years," she said, "Long enough."

With this contract in mind, subsequent sessions entailed a searching for the etiology or inception of the point at which dysfunction took priority over growth. The movement therapy sessions became a series of microcosms in which to try out more adaptive behavior to be integrated into her experience of being-in-the-world.

### Mark

Mark was a member of an ongoing dance-movement therapy group of functioning, motivated young adults. Prior to the session described below he had been working on various pre-adolescent developmental tasks. However, it was during an intensive ritual experience that much of his process came to fruition and was organized. The following represents his phenomenological experience of his rite of passage from puberty into manhood.

At first, he described his experience as one of boredom—not knowing what he should do. He felt he wanted to hide in some way and shrouded himself with a large black piece of material and waited. Then Mark related a sense of the present reality fading. He stated, "I began to realize why I was there . . . was that I was a chieftan's son and this was my day of becoming. I had to prove myself—that I could be a man."

Mark said he had felt foolish. When his sense of silliness subsided he felt a realization come to him in its entirety. "What I had to do was kill the beast and capture a woman. It was a realization like, 'Oh, that's why I'm sitting here. I'm sitting here preparing for that,' " Mark related with some liveliness.

He became more serious. "The thing I'm most in touch with is that there was this overwhelming sense of importance; that I had to do it because a lot was riding on it."

Before he began his quest, he described killing the boy in him. He did this by having the black cape represent his boy. He danced centrifugal spiraling circles around it. His movement became freer and at last he released himself from his relationship to the cape/boy. He then related a sense of "stalking out his territory." His movements had vertical assertive qualities to them as he confronted other group members who related to him from their own psyches unknowing that they were to serve as various archetypes for him.

The wild beast[5] (another male group member) approached him grabbing and pulling at his cape. At first Mark let himself be dragged about the room. When he attempted to use strength, he was overpowered by other group members. Then he realized he would have to use guile or trickery. Mark related, "It required thinking, planning and watching for the right moment."

Then the woman appeared in the rite. She was a group member with whom Mark had had a special personal connection. She danced around them in weight and flow with her pelvis initiating the movement. Mark relates, "I felt like we fought over her to a standstill, then after a rest, fought again." But finally Mark's guile won out, he completely entwined the beast in a long stretch cloth. The three of them with the beast in the middle, still wrapped up, began prancing around the periphery of the other group members. They then collapsed on the floor. Mark separated himself and sat erect facing them. He related his presenting the beast and the woman to his father (yet another group member who unknowingly was participating in Mark's ritual). Mark commented, "Initially I was a proud swaggering kind of warrior, a very animal-brute kind of warrior—almost totally instinctual; just wanting to boast and establish my territory. After capturing the beast and woman there was a feeling of maturity. I was still a man, I was still victorious, but I felt bigger in stature and had gotten rid of the need to boast." The experience was

5. Of interest to note here is that the man who Mark had given the personification of the wild beast was engaged in his own unconscious fantasy. Mark, in turn represented some other symbolic aspect to him.

discussed in the context of Mark's life: his childhood, his recent past, related dreams, his present, and his future path.

In finishing, Mark commented, "In some way or other, everything that I've done since I had the choice, that is, since I left home and took responsibility for myself, has had the quality of a search for something. I'm not sure what I'm looking for, but somehow there seems to be something sacred about the looking. There is something in the looking that provides meaning for me, that provides purpose. So maybe that's what sacred *is*: that which provides purpose and meaning. Without that, there would be no point to my life."

Mark, without knowing it, had undergone a classic archetypal male puberty ritual. Joseph Campbell,[6] Carl Jung,[7] and other psycho/anthropologists have characterized this universal cross-cultural ritual process: For a boy to become a man he must first separate himself from his boyhood, his personal mother, and the archetypal great mother as well, in order to develop consciousness distinct from the unconscious. From there he enters a luminous period in which he is neither boy nor man. In this initiation-transition phase he must subdue the beasts of his primitive drives and enter into a mystical marriage between the hero as soul knower and master—and the woman as anima, natural organic flow, and the unconscious. Both the masculine and feminine aspects of Mark's psychology were integrated through movement interactions with these projected personifications of his psychology. In the final reunion-transformation phase, he is released from the confines of the father complex through completion of the tasks and receives the boon which serves to shed light on manly wisdom and provide a bridge to his feminine side, his anima.

### Diane

At 27, Diane had a strong heronic athletic body. In her initial session as a private client she was dressed in a jogging outfit through which her developed muscles could easily be delineated. I was dwarfed by her physical size. Her amazon-like body, however, was juxtaposed by the face of a little girl. Her curly flaxen hair provided a braided frame to her soft pretty face. Her clear blue eyes projected sadness and fear, and a yearning to be accepted.

She moved with directness and intention. Her muscular armor encapsulated much of her potential free flow, however, probably "protecting" the rest of the little girl within her.

Diane was the only daughter and oldest of three children. She described her mother as cold and her father as creative but unexpressive. She remembered spending her latency playing with her brothers and the boys in the

6. Joseph Campbell, *Hero with a Thousand Faces*. (New York: World Publishing Co., 1970.)
7. Carl Jung, *Memories, Dreams, and Reflections*. (New York: Random House, 1961.)

neighborhood. Puberty and adolescence were emotionally painful. She recalls consciously trying to delay puberty, pressing her hands against her blossoming breasts in hope that they would cease to develop. Her pain and confusion culminated at 19 when she institutionalized herself in a private psychiatric facility for 9 months.

She subsequently finished college and began working as a sports instructor. She had been married a year prior to a man who she said, "has softer skin than I."

What had brought her to see me? She replied that during her stay in the hospital it was dance therapy that had provided her with special avenues in her journey. "Movement can cut through places I can talk around," she said. She had heard of me and felt that she wanted to begin to work again. She felt ready, although she wasn't quite sure for what.

In her second session Diane spoke of an injury to her coccyx which had occurred soon after her marriage and was acting up again. This injury was not by accident, and neither was it by chance that it was exacerbated upon her reentrance into therapy. It was part of her that refused to go unnoticed. Focusing on the area, she described it as being dark on the outside and light in the middle. Gradually an entrapped dancing fairy came into focus in its core. It was a month before this spirit could be explored, as she feared that it was bad or evil. In processing this experience she began to be aware that she had introjected her parents' values and behaviors to sexuality.

Her need to do what the authority figure says and her hidden rage emerged in the transference during the third session. I had suggested that she allow a metaphoric improvisation that she was exploring in her hand to extend into her body. A battle ensued within her body, creating bound tension along with disassociated and distorted flow. We explored her conflict in terms of its somatic manifestations, the therapeutic relationship, and in relation to her parents.

In the next session she brought in a poem which reflected her view of water as the "power source." Paying credence to her negative authority transference, I suggested that she allow herself to be in this water in some way, and this brought a simple but significant experience to Diane. After silent tears, she reflected, "I feel connected . . . my mind and my body." Though ephemerial, it was a first for her since her early childhood.

It was Halloween and she was dressed in black. She wanted to be a magician-sorceress. She had brought in a picture of the dance spirit and felt she could now contact it.

Diane began to move. At first it appeared that her ego was directing her. After a cut on the record of water sounds, she emerged in authentic movement. Posture-gesture merger occurred in flow. It was as if she was being moved into the "spirit realms." After she had gently come "down to earth" she described going to each person she cared about and giving them love.

In her last fall session before her winter ski season, she became increasingly aware of how other peoples' "shoulds," at work and in the past with her parents, kept her from experiencing herself. During movement active imagination her legs and arms writhed in bound wringing patterns. She later depicted this experience as a figure with arms and legs curled inward as if in retroflected expression.

Therapy resumed in the spirng, and with it a more positive transference emerged. Through simply creating space for authentic movement (Whitehouse, 1979), she had the following experience:

Her torso, resting at first, gradually began to move. The pattern was strong and bound, originating centrally from her back, and her breathing was clearly in synchrony with her movements. Those effort qualities soon subsided, and free flow and lightness emerged. When the experience reached a natural closing she felt deeply appreciative for the time and space to be "touched" by her inside. At first she described some part of her saying, "Do something to get them off your back," i.e., all those she viewed as authority figures. She experienced surrendering and going deeper, and began to imagine a beautiful woman running with gentle lightness in a field. A three- or four-year-old girl came into focus. She was very feminine with curls and a fancy dress. The woman took the girl's hand then and helped her pick flowers. It became clear to me that the little girl reflected in her face and the little girl of this image were one and the same. This appeared to be where her development was arrested. Further discussion regarding the birth of her brother and her father's relationship to her during the oedipal phase confirmed the assumption.

Subsequently a transference dream emerged. In it I am having all my clients over for dinner. I am preparing the meal while Diane talks quietly with her fellow clients. She feels comfortable. She remarks that she came to the dinner from one direction and will leave by another. After hearing this dream she was able to remember her mother taking her to barber shops to have her hair cut and that she continuously bought her clothes and shoes two sizes too big, and always from boys' departments. Diane related how uncomfortable she felt with other girls, feeling that they made fun of her and played "other games" with the boys.

Upon request, she brought in a picture of herself at four years of age. She recalled her father saying to her as an older child, "What happened to our happy little girl?" Diane said she couldn't connect to this pretty, contented little girl, but recalled herself at around six feeling deeply lonely and wondering what she had done wrong. Neither her father nor mother could accept her awakening feminine sexuality.

The climax of her deepening awareness came when she was discussing her trying out for a male-dominated team. She said, "I'm afraid they're going to find out . . . I'm embarrassed that they're going to find out I'm a woman." I quietly remarked that that was an important insight.

The following week she was furious with me. Why hadn't I protected her from the pain of it all. She had become aware that everything she did, from being with her husband to "taking out the garbage," was imbued with "trying to keep people from finding out."

In the next session she brought in a couple dreams. In the first one she goes to the basement and finds that her father has a ski shop. He gives her some magical old cross-country skis. The next dream has her skiing with a man who is the paragon of manhood, and she is equal to his prowess.

In a movement exploration Diane walked around the room with the skis her father had given her. She gradually became more facile. She stopped and moved to the center of the room. For the first time I saw the muscular athletic armor of her body soften as if it were sloughed away. Her demeanor and posture became that of a little girl. She cried softly. She said that this was a gift of love connection from her father and she knew she would come to use these skis well. I reminded her that in her last dream, she, very much a woman, was no longer secondary to the male, but was his equal.

In a subsequent session Diane was able to move toward me, sobbing, and put her head into my lap. In the past she had always felt "funny" being alone with women, undoubtedly in part due to fears of latent homosexuality. She said later how important it was for her to be able to receive from me, another woman. I clarified that it was nice to be able to receive love from another woman without sexual issues being added to the experience. She nodded in affirmation.

Through her movement reenactments of her maladaptive environment, as well as through her explorations of the adaptive oedipal tasks of a four- to five-year-old in relationship to her father, mother, and myself as transferential object, she was able to allow a positive feminine figure to emerge from her unconscious. In the next sessions she brought in several pictures of herself. She said they reminded her of me. This figure represented part of her feminine psychodevelopment which was now being integrated.

In her last session (she was moving West) she described how initially she hadn't known why she was re-entering movement therapy, but had begun to understand that she needed to rediscover and accept her womanhood. She described how her interpersonal relationships with other women had changed, how she had become more comfortable being "one of the girls." The integration of the oedipal inner genital phase and related efforts of lightness and flow had helped her in her involvement in sports.

She also mentioned how she was beginning to integrate our relationship into her work. She had begun teaching women to ski in a program entitled "Woman's Way." Through this method women would utilize their intuitive relationship to nature and its timing in their skiing, just as she was beginning to do in her life.

## CHAPTER X

# Conclusion

Now, after you have read through this text, digest what makes sense to you—what feels right—and disregard the rest. Each therapist is going to work just a little bit differently from the one next to him—a highly favorable situation in the author's opinion. What is not needed in this or any other field are programmed robots moving and responding in identical, totally predetermined patterns.

This book is meant to give the reader a taste of how one person sees the relationship between one philosophical approach and one modality. All of what has been written here "feels right" to the author. She has seen it work enough times to feel it worthwhile to pass it on. It is hoped that this book will be one of many resource books which are used when brainstorming is needed. It is not meant to be a blinder to anyone's creative process. The suggested movement activities are only examples from a myriad of experiences which could be used. By others thoughts with the ideas expressed here, creativity can be exercised, not suppressed.

Neither is this book meant to stifle spontaniety and "here and now" reactions to "here and now" situations. Going into a therapy session with a head filled with specific exercises, goals, etc., is perhaps one of the worst possible mistakes a therapist can make. This situation only serves to desensitize the therapist to where the client is and how he feels at that moment. It is not meant to suggest either that a therapist ignore the direction that he and the client both feel they should work toward. However, there is an optimal compromise: one in which the therapist reacts to the "here and now" of where his client is such that he could duplicate the mood tone from his own feelings if needed in order to sense the person with whom he is working. The "treatment plan," then, is placed in reserve or subliminal awareness, if you will, far enough away so that it only comes to the forefront when needed.

Ideally, however, there would be no necessity for even an occasional calling forth of such data. If this information is truly integrated, it will flow within the breath pulse of the movement therapist in spontaneous client-centered movement interactions.

# APPENDIX

Developmental Chart

*Ego Psychology,* Jungian Analytic Psychology, and Related Developmental Constellations

Gesell, Piaget, and Effort-Shape Developmental Correlation

Levels of Organization Form for Dance-Movement Therapy

Maladaptive Behavior Evaluation Form

Outline for Movement Profile

| CONSTELLATIONS | 0-1 mons. | 1-6 mons. | | 6 mons.-1 yr. | 1-1½ yrs. | 1½-2 yrs. | 2-3 yrs. | 3-4 yrs. |
|---|---|---|---|---|---|---|---|---|
| Flow of Breath | Normal Breath Flow | | | | | | | |
| Effort | Primal Regulation of Tension Flow | | | Spacial Pre-effort | Weight Pre-effort | | Time Pre-effort | |
| Shape | Symmetrical and Asymmetrical Shape Flow | | | Horizontal Directional Shape | Vertical Directional Shape | | Sagittal Directional Shape | |
| Posture-Gesture | P-G Flow | | | | | | | |
| Flow Rhythms | Oral Libidinal | | | Oral Aggressive | Anal Libidinal | Anal Sadistic | Urethral Libidinal | Urethral Sadistic |
| Body-Image | | | Positive Affect in Self | Body, Body Part Relationship; Body Differentiate from Environment | | Movement of the Body Through Space | | |
| Drive-Object | | Libidinal Self Investment | External Libidinal Investment | Investment in Aggressive Drive in External Object | | | | |
| Dyadic | | Ego-Centric | Object-Dependent | | Object-Ambivalent | | Semi-Autonomous | |
| GROUP | One-to-One | | | | | | Parallel | Task |
| RITES OF PASSAGE | Birth Ritual Process | Weaning Ritual Process | | | | | | |
| TACTILE PERCEPTION | | Recognition | Discriminate | | Recall | | | |
| KINESTHETIC PERCEPTION | | Recognition | Discriminate | | Recall | | | |
| VESTIBULAR PERCEPTION | | Recognition | Discriminate | | Recall | | | |
| COGNITIVE REPRESENTATION | | Enactive | | | | | Iconic | |
| THOUGHT PROCESS | Primary Process | | | | | Secondary Process | | |
| PLAY-WORK | | | | | | | | |

| 4-5 | 5-6 | 6-7 | 7-8 | 8-9 | 9-10 | 10-11 | 11-12 | 12-15 | 15-18 | 18-20 | 35 | 65- | |
|---|---|---|---|---|---|---|---|---|---|---|---|---|---|
| Space Effort | Weight Effort | Temporal Effort | | 2 Effort Combination | | | | 3 Effort Combination | | | | | |
| Horizontal Shaping | Vertical Shaping | Sagittal Shaping | | 2 Shape Combination | | | | 3 Shape Combination | | | | | |
| Effort-Shape Gesture Mergers | | | | | | | | E-S P-G Mergers | | | | | |
| Feminine Libidinal Aggressive | Phallic Libidinal Aggressive | | | | | | | Phallic-Feminine | | | | | |
| Sexual Identity | | | | | | | | | | | Aging Process | | |
| | | | | | | | | | | | | | |
| | | | Chumship | | | | | | Autonomous | | | | |
| | Ego-Centric Cooperative | | | | | | | | | | | | |
| | | | | | | Puberty Ritual Process | | | | Marriage Ritual Process | Parenthood Ritual Process | Retirement Ritual Process | Dying Ritual Process |
| | | | | | | | | | | | | | |
| | | | | | | | | | | | | | |
| Iconic | | | | | | | | Abstract | | | | | |
| Secondary Process | | | | | | | | | Tertiary Process | | Quaternary Process | | |
| | | | | | | | Dance as Hobby | | Dance as Occupation | | | | |

| | Ego Psychology Eric Erikson's Eight Stages | Related Developmental Constellations | Jungian Analytic Psychology Erich Neumann |
|---|---|---|---|
| 0–18 mo. | *Trust*<br>vs.<br>*Mistrust*<br>Oral<br>Sensori | Egocentric, one-to-one<br>Positive libidinal investment in self<br>Oral libidinal, oral aggressive<br>Spatial pre-efforts<br>Horizontal directional shape<br>Primary process<br>Birth Ritual process | *Post-Natal Embryonic Phase*<br>Primary unitary relationship<br>Social uterine phase<br>Ego dormant in uroboros<br>Participation mystique<br>Self externalized in mother<br>Experience of personality on a body level |
| 18 mo.–2½ | *Autonomy*<br>vs.<br>*Shame & Doubt*<br>Anal<br>Muscular | Object ambivalent & semi-autonomous<br>Parallel group<br>Anal libidinal, anal sadistic<br>Gravitational pre-efforts<br>Vertical directional shape | *Second Matriarchal Phase*<br>Separation of World Parents—<br>Polarization of world into opposites<br>Internal ego achieves central position |
| 2½–5½ | *Initiative*<br>vs.<br>*Guilt*<br>Locomotive<br>Genital | Task group<br>Urethral libidinal, urethral sadistic<br>Phallic libidinal, phallic sadistic (outer genital)<br>Inner genital libidinal & sadistic<br>Time pre-efforts<br>Sagittal directional shape<br>Sexual identity<br>Weaning ritual process<br>Secondary process | *Phallic-Chthonian Stage of Ego*<br>Vegetative-passive: 2½–3½<br>Animal-body motility: 3½–4½<br>Phallus-symbol of autonomy of unconscious and body<br>Ego activities dependent on body experience<br>*Magical Warlike Stage of Ego*<br>Ego opposes mother<br>Consciousness of the masculine |

| | Ego Psychology Eric Erikson's Eight Stages | Related Developmental Constellations | Jungian Analytic Psychology Erick Neumann |
|---|---|---|---|
| 5½-12 | *Industry* vs. *Inferiority*<br>Latency | Chumship relationship<br>Egocentric cooperative group<br>Space, weight, time efforts<br>Horizontal, vertical, sagittal shapes<br>2-Effort & shape combinations | *Patriarchate Magic Warlike Stage of Ego*<br>Father replaces mother as superego |
| 12-20 | *Identity* vs. *Role Confusion*<br>Puberty Adolescence | Phallic-Inner Genital<br>(Genital) rhythm<br>3-Effort Combination<br>3-Shape Combination<br>E-S P-G mergers<br>Puberty ritual process<br>Tertiary process | *Solar-Warlike Phase of Ego*<br>Power based on magical connection with the Light<br>Males—receive masculine via identification—spiritual mysteries<br>Females—receive masculine via penetration of the soul with the numinous—nature mysteries |
| 20-35 | *Intimacy* vs. *Isolation*<br>Young Adulthood | Marriage ritual<br>Autonomous relationship<br>Parenthood ritual process | *Solar Rational Ego Stage*<br>Ego's concern to adapt to external reality<br>Ego—primary reality<br>Ego adapts to society & consciousness |
| 35— | *Generativity* vs. *Stagnation*<br>Adulthood<br>*Integrity* vs. *Despair* | Aging Process<br>Quaternary Process<br>Retirement ritual process<br>Dying ritual process | *Shift to Self Stage*<br>Self replaces ego in primacy<br>Contact with transpersonal thou<br>Contact with collective unconscious |

## GESELL, PIAGET AND EFFORT-SHAPE DEVELOPMENTAL CONSTELLATION

| Age | Effort | Shape |
|---|---|---|
| 0–1 mo. | Primal regulation of tension flow<br><br>Ability to initiate, continue, and cessate free and bound flow interchanges. | Symmetrical and asymmetrical shape flow<br><br>Alternation of bipolar growing and shrinking and ability to shape in a unipolar relationship to the environment. |
| 6–9 mo.<br><br>9–12 mo. | Spacial pre-effort<br>Ability to channel and be flexible | Horizontal directional shape<br>Ability to shape sideways and across the body<br>Communication |
| 1½–2½ | Gravitation or weight pre-effort<br>Ability to move with vehemence and gentility | Vertical directional shape<br>Ability to shape upwards and downwards<br>Presentation |
| 2½–3<br>3–4 | Time pre-effort<br>Ability to move with suddenness and hesitation | Sagittal directional shape<br>Ability to shape forwards and backwards<br>Operation |

| Piaget | Gesell |
|---|---|
| Sensori-motor: Reflex stage<br>Hereditary organic reflexes<br>Sucking and grasping | Grasp reflex<br>Sucking reflex |
| Sensori-motor: Primary circular reactions<br>First acquired adaptations<br>Concepts of groups and reversibility without mental representation<br>Voluntary movements | Grasp reflex lost; raises head<br>Initiates arm in grasping object<br>Clutches |
| Sensori-motor: Secondary circular reactions<br>Movement centered on maintaining results produced in environment<br>Intentional adaptations<br>Foresight and incipient goal directed behavior | Assumes crawling posture<br>Creeps<br>Transfers object from hand to hand |
| Sensori-motor: Coordination of secondary schema<br>Emergence of means end relationship<br>Beginning of sign understanding<br>Concept of object permanence | Sits<br>Brings two objects together |
| Sensori-motor: Tertiary circular reactions<br>Stabilization of object permanence<br>Discovery of new means through active experimentation | Cruses with support<br>Crude release<br>Pincer grasp |
| Sensori-motor: Inventions of new means through mental combinations<br>Internatlization of sensori-motor schema<br>Use of foresight in solving sensorimotor problems | Walks without support<br>Fine manipulative skill |
| Pre-operational I: Pre-conceptual substage<br>Extracting concepts from sensory experiences<br>Language-verbal communication<br>Presentation and representation of objects<br>Transduction—reasoning from particular to particular without generalization<br>Syncretism—linking of unrelated material<br>Realism—illegitimate generalization<br>Artificialism—belief that natural events are caused by humans<br>Egocentrism in language and thought | Runs<br>Regards and reaches simultaneously |
| | Up and down stairs<br>Jumps down 12 inches<br>Stands on one foot |
| | Runs smoothly at different speeds<br>Alternates progression in climbing |

| Age | Effort | Shape |
|---|---|---|
| 4–5 | Spacial effort<br>Ability to move with directness and indirectness | Horizontal shaping<br>Ability to shape in the horizontal plane with spreading and enclosing movements |
| 5–6 | Gravitational or weight effort<br>Ability to move with strength and lightness | Vertical shaping<br>Ability to shape in the vertical plane with ascending and descending movements |
| 6–7 | Time efforts<br>Ability to move with acceleration or quickness and deceleration or slowness | Sagittal shaping<br>Ability to shape in the sagittal plane with advancing and retreating movements |
| 8–12 | Inner attitudes—2-effort combinations<br>Movement involving temporal-spacial, spacial-gravitational, and temporal-gravitational factors | 2 Shaping combinations<br>Movement involving horizontal-vertical, horizontal-sagittal, and vertical-sagittal shaping factors |
| 12–15 | Full efforts—3-effort combinations<br>Ability to float, glide, dab, flick, press, wring, slash, punch | 3 Shaping combinations<br>Movement involving attributes from each of the three planes: horizontal, sagittal,and vertical |

| Piaget | Gesell |
|---|---|
| Pre-operational II: Intuitive Substage<br>Manipulation of experimental objects more effectively<br>Cannot yet consider two or more dimensions at the same time, but focuses on one aspect at a time | Long swinging steps<br>Stops and goes quickly<br>Throws overhead |
| | Walks on toes<br>Climbs and skips<br>Narrow symmetrical controlled motions<br>Grasping coordination |
| | Constant activity<br>Approaches activity with more abandon and/or deliberation<br>Interest in stunts and tools |
| Concrete Operations<br>Operational stage in logical thinking<br>Groupings of operations using: conservation, associativity, identity, reversibility, substitution, multiplication of classes and series, and tree of classes<br>Emergence of grouping of combinations | Repeat skills to master<br>Timing under better control<br>Competitive sports<br>Handwriting a tool |
| Formal Operations<br>Combination of operations and schema<br>Abstract thought<br>Ability to deal with a wide variety of complex relations (e.g., ability to move using all possible combinations of effort-shape attributes)<br>Formulation of assumptions and hypotheses<br>Reflective thinking<br>Concepts of continuity, infinity, symbolism | Learns hobby and job skills<br>Copes with environment using gross and fine motor skills |

Name: ______________________________ Age: _____ Date: ___________

I. History
   A. Vital statistics
   B. Childhood to present
   C. Family system
   D. Work history
   E. Medical history and precautions
   F. Diagnosis
   G. Medication

II. Referral

III. Time, date, and under what circumstances observations made

IV. Characteristic Body Attitude, Movement Profile, and Summary:

V. Prognosis and recommendations

## LEVELS OF ORGANIZATION FORM FOR DANCE-MOVEMENT THERAPY

Penny Bernstein, Ph.D. OTR, DTR

Flow of Breath

1. Breath flow ______ [ ]
2. Breathing in the service of movement ______ [ ]

Effort Levels of Organization

1. Primal regulation of tension flow ______ [ ]
2. Spatial pre-effort ______ [ ]
3. Gravitational pre-effort ______ [ ]
4. Temporal pre-effort ______ [ ]
5. Spatial effort ______ [ ]
6. Gravitational effort ______ [ ]
7. Temporal effort ______ [ ]
8. Inner attitudes (2-effort combination) ______ [ ]
9. Full efforts (3-effort combination) ______ [ ]

Shape levels of Organization

1. Symmetrical shape flow ______ [ ]
2. Asymmetrical shape flow ______ [ ]
3. Horizontal directional shape ______ [ ]
4. Vertical directional shape ______ [ ]
5. Sagittal directional shape ______ [ ]
6. Horizontal shaping ______ [ ]
7. Vertical shaping ______ [ ]

8. Sagittal shaping
9. 2-shape combination
10. 3-shape combination

Posture-Gesture Levels of Organization

1. Posture-gesture flow
2. Merging of gesture systems
3. Merging of posture-gesture systems

Tension Flow Rhythms Levels of Organization

1. Oral libidinal
2. Oral aggressive
3. Anal libidinal
4. Anal sadistic
5. Urethral libidinal
6. Urethral sadistic
7. Inner genital libidinal
8. Inner genital sadistic
9. Phallic (outer genital) libidinal
10. Phallic (outer genital) Sadistic
11. Phallic-inner genital (genital adult)

Body-Image Levels of Organization

1. Investment of positive affect in body
2. Differentiation of body from the environment
3. Recognition of the body parts and their relationship

| | |
|---|---|
| 4. Movement of the body through space | |
| 5. Sexual identity | |
| 6. Aging Process | |
| Drive-Object Levels of Organization | |
| 1. Investment of libidinal drive in self | |
| 2. Investment of libidinal drive in external objects | |
| 3. Investment of aggressive drive in external objects | |
| Dyadic Levels Organizaton | |
| 1. Egocentric—symbiotic | |
| 2. Object-dependent—(Practicing) Separation-Individuation | |
| 3. Object-ambivalent (Rapprochement) Separation-Individuation | |
| 4. Semi-autonomous | |
| 5. Chumship—Object Constancy | |
| 6. Autonomous | |
| Group Levels of Organization | |
| 1. One-to-one | |
| 2. Parallel | |
| 3. Task | |
| 4. Ego-centric and group cooperative | |
| Rites of Passage Levels of Organization | |
| 1. Birth Ritual Process | |
| 2. Weaning Ritual Process | |
| 3. Puberty Ritual Process | |

| | |
|---|---|
| 4. Marriage Ritual Process | |
| 5. Parenthood Ritual Process | |
| 6. Retirement Ritual Process | |
| 7. Dying Ritual Process | |
| Tactile Perceptual Levels of Organization | |
| 1. Tactile recognition | |
| 2. Tactile discrimination | |
| 3. Tactile retention and recall | |
| Kinesthetic Perceptual Levels of Organization | |
| 1. Kinesthetic recognition | |
| 2. Kinesthetic discrimination | |
| 3. Kinesthetic retention and recall | |
| Vestibular Perceptual Levels of Organization | |
| 1. Vestibular recognition | |
| 2. Vestibular discrimination | |
| 3. Vestibular retention and recall | |
| Cognitive Representation Levels of Organization | |
| 1. Enactive | |
| 2. Iconic | |
| 3. Abstract | |
| Thought Processes Levels of Organization | |
| 1. Primary process | |
| 2. Secondary process | |
| 3. Tertiary process | |
| 4. Quaternary process | |

Play-Work Levels of Organization

| | |
|---|---|
| 1. Dance as a hobby | |
| 2. Dance as an occupation | |

## MALADAPTIVE BEHAVIOR DANCE-MOVEMENT THERAPY EVALUATION FORM

Penny Bernstein, Ph.D. OTR, DTR

| | |
|---|---|
| **Flow of Breath** | |
| 1. Breathing shallow and below normal | |
| 2. Hypernea | |
| 3. Air sucked in | |
| 4. Vertical breath pattern | |
| 5. Breath held | |
| 6. Decreased breath rate | |
| 7. Immobilization of chest | |
| 8. Immobilization of diaphragm | |
| 9. Immobilization of pelvis | |
| 10. Immobilization of abdomen | |
| 11. Flaccid-limp | |
| 12. Body or body part muscular rigidity, "dead spots" | |
| 13. Mute | |
| 14. Shallow vocalization | |
| 15. Rapid speech | |
| 16. Slow speech | |
| **Effort Levels of Organization** | |
| 1. Inability to distinguish movement continuity/discontinuity | |
| 2. Lack of an adaptive range of tension flow variations | |
| 3. Dominance or excessive bound flow | |
| 4. Dominance or excessive free flow | |

| | |
|---|---|
| 5. Dominance of neutral flow | |
| 6. Difficulty in adaptive usage of channeling | |
| 7. Difficulty in adaptive usage of flexibility | |
| 8. Difficulty in adaptive usage of vehemence | |
| 9. Difficulty in adaptive usage of gentleness | |
| 10. Difficulty in adaptive usage of hesitation | |
| 11. Difficulty in adaptive usage of suddenness | |
| 12. Dominant pre-effort motor apparatus for defense mechanisms | |
| 13. Defense mechanisms used: | |
| | |
| | |
| | |
| 14. Difficulty in adaptive usage of directness | |
| 15. Difficulty in adaptive usage of indirectness | |
| 16. Lack of adequate ability to investigate or define | |
| 17. Difficulty in adaptive usage of lightness | |
| 18. Difficulty in adaptive usage of strength | |
| 19. Lack of adequate ability to utilize determination, persistence, conviction, and/or firmness or purpose | |
| 20. Difficulty in adaptive usage of slowness | |
| 21. Difficulty in adaptive usage of quickness | |
| 22. Lack of an adequate sense of timing or decisiveness | |
| 23. Postural efforts dashing with gestural efforts | |
| 24. Presence of punitive superego | |

| | |
|---|---|
| 25. Difficulty in adaptive use of a two-effort quality | |
| 26. Unadaptive exaggeration of an inner attitude: | |
| | |
| | |
| | |
| 27. Difficulty in adaptively utilizing a 3-effort combination | |
| 28. Absence of indulging efforts | |
| 29. Absence of fighting efforts | |
| 30. Clashes between pre-efforts and efforts | |
| 31. Diffuse effort phrases | |
| Shape Levels of Organization | |
| 1. Difficulty in adaptive usage of symmetrical shape flow | |
| 2. Excessive bound bulging: feelings of bursting with anger | |
| 3. Excessive bound lengthening: rage and/or anxiety stage | |
| 4. Excessive bound widening: fear of falling apart | |
| 5. Excessive bound hollowing: feelings of being knotted up | |
| 6. Excessive bound shortening: feelings of being wound up | |
| 7. Excessive bound narrowing: feelings of emptiness | |
| 8. Predominance of hollowing, shortening, and/or narrowing | |
| 9. Predominance of bulging, lengthening, and/or widening | |
| 10. Difficulty in the transfer of libidinal impulses from self to other | |
| 11. Difficulty in the transfer of aggressive impulses from self to other | |
| 12. Difficulty in relating to the inner space of the body | |

13. Bizarre, manneristic shaping
14. Difficulty in adaptive usage of asymmetrical shape flow
15. Continuous maladaptive asymmetrical body stance
16. Lack of reaction to a discrete stimulus
17. Inappropriate movement response to positive and/or negative stimulus
18. Difficulty in adaptive usage of sideways direction
19. Difficulty in adaptive usage of movement across the body
20. Difficulty in adaptive usage of upwards direction
21. Difficulty in adaptive usage of downwards direction
22. Difficulty in adaptive usage of forward direction
23. Difficulty in adaptive usage of backward direction
24. Defends against object(s)
25. Difficulty with adaptive use of spreading
26. Difficulty in adaptive usage of enclosing
27. Lack of an adequate awareness of the range of possibilities or the ability to explore
28. Difficulty in adaptive usage of ascending
29. Difficulty in adaptive usage of descending
30. Lack of an adequate ability to confront
31. Difficulty in adaptive usage of advancing
32. Difficulty in adaptive usage of retreating
33. Lack of an adequate sense of anticipation, farsightedness, and sense of the effects of the present in relation to the future

| | |
|---|---|
| 34. Lack of presence of motor apparatus for complex object relationships | |
| 35. Low self appraisal | |
| 36. Conflict between gestural shaping and postural shaping | |
| 37. Denigration of self in relation to objects | |
| 38. Difficulty in adaptive usage of 2-shape combinations | |
| 39. Difficulty in adaptive usage of 3-shape combinations | |
| 40. Clashes between directional shape and shaping | |
| 41. Clashes between shape flow and shaping | |
| 42. Fragmented shape phrases | |
| 43. Diffuse shape phrases | |
| **Effort-Shape Relationship** | |
| 1. Difficulty in appropriate effort-shape combination | |
| 2. Presence of intrasystemic ego conflict; specify E-S mismatching: | |
| | |
| | |
| | |
| 3. Inter-systemic id-ego-superego conflict, specify rhythms, E-S mismatching: | |
| | |
| | |
| | |
| **Posture-Gesture Levels of Organization** | |
| 1. Difficulty in adaptive flow variation in postures | |
| 2. Difficulty in E-S flow P-G mergers | |
| 3. Difficulty in adaptive E-S G mergers | |

| | |
|---|---|
| 4. Difficulty in E-S G-P or P-G mergers | |
| 5. Gestures unrelated to postures (or vice-versa) | |
| 6. Artificial movements (diminished postural adjustments) | |
| 7. Doll-like or puppet-like movements | |
| 8. Idiosyncratic bizarre movements as compensation for inability to merge | |
| 9. Predominance of inadaptive peripheral gestures | |
| 10. Lack of adaptibility of postures | |
| 11. Lack of posturally expressed affect | |
| 12. Exaggeration of movements | |
| 13. Fleeting postural movement | |
| 14. Presence of only single phases of postural movement | |
| 15. No successive postural movement in limbs | |
| Tension Flow Rhythm Levels of Organization | |
| 1. Insufficient amount of oral rhythms | |
| 2. Excessive amount of oral rhythms | |
| 3. Continuous and/or diffuse crying | |
| 4. Vomiting or nausea | |
| 5. Tense deep neck muscles; upper back | |
| 6. Back arched, stiffening, resistance of arm and leg extension | |
| 7. Insufficient amount of oral aggressive rhythms | |
| 8. Excessive amount of oral aggressive rhythms | |
| 9. Tense throat, jaw, chest, eyes | |
| 10. Restless grasping | |
| 11. Blowing, spitting, biting | |

| | |
|---|---|
| 12. Insufficient amount of anal rhythms | |
| 13. Excessive amount of anal rhythms | |
| 14. Continuous kicking and slapping | |
| 15. Insufficient amount of anal sadistic rhythms | |
| 16. Excessive amount of anal sadistic rhythms | |
| 17. Retroflexed anal sadistic rhythms | |
| 18. Tense buttocks, thighs, calves, and shoulders | |
| 19. Pelvis tilted forward; upward | |
| 20. Insufficient amount of urethral rhythms | |
| 21. Excessive amount of urethral rhythms | |
| 22. Flowing everywhere with little control | |
| 23. Insufficient amount of urethral sadistic rhythms | |
| 24. Excessive amount of urethral sadistic rhythms | |
| 25. Tense lower pelvis | |
| 26. Insufficient amount of inner genital rhythms | |
| 27. Excessive amount of inner genital rhythms | |
| 28. Insufficient amount of inner genital sadistic rhythms | |
| 29. Excessive amount of inner genital sadistic rhythms | |
| 30. Insufficient amount of outer genital rhythms (phallic) | |
| 31. Excessive amount of outer genital rhythms (phallic) | |
| 32. Insufficient amount of outer genital sadistic rhythms (phallic) | |
| 33. Excessive amount of outer genital sadistic rhythms (phallic) | |
| 34. Inappropriate oedipal resolution | |

35. Insufficient amount of adult genital rhythms
36. Excessive mixture of o, a, or u rhythms with others
37. Lack of presence of phrase-appropriate pure rhythms
38. Lack of drive differentiation; specify:
39. Fragmentation of rhythms

Body-Image Levels of Organization

1. Negative B-I
2. Unkempt clothes, poor hygenic care
3. Self mutilation, suicidal ideation
4. Difficulty in adaptively differentiating the body from the environment
5. Body boundaries lack adaptive bound flow and shrinking in shape flow
6. Fear of dismemberment
7. Individual merges with objects
8. Difficulty in recognizing and identifying body parts
9. Difficulty in recognizing body part relationships
10. Difficulty in differentiating internal from external
11. B-I distortions: size, shape, absence, presence
12. Difficulty in moving through space
13. Difficulty in adaptive motor planning
14. Laterality dominance and/or inadequate reciprocal movement
15. Insufficient amount of genital rhythms
16. Bound pelvis

17. Lack of body conditioning
18. Denial of aging
19. Puer or puella aeternus complex

Drive-Object Levels of Organization

1. Inappropriate inhibition of libidinal rhythms
2. Insufficient amount of indulging pre-efforts
3. Difficulty in the adaptive use of indulging efforts and corresponding shape
4. Difficulty in adaptive use of fighting efforts, pre-efforts, and corresponding shape
5. Lack of postural merger of aggression
6. Denial of anger
7. Fear of letting go
8. Diffuse, non-directed anger, i.e., no use of space
9. Difficulty in the use of strength when expressing anger
10. Difficulty in the use of quickness when expressing anger
11. Lack of aggressive movements when confronted with an aggressive object
12. Splitting object relationship

Dyadic Levels of Organization

1. Autistic deanimated relationship with therapist
2. Inability in merging movement pattern with therapist
3. Difficulty in formulating a trust relationship
4. Inability to make use of therapist as symbiotic buffer
5. Difficulty in differentiating from primary object
6. Difficulty in self-initiating or cessating movement

| | |
|---|---|
| 7. Inappropriate negative response to authority figure | |
| 8. Over-dependent relationship with therapist | |
| 9. Inability to satisfy the needs of another | |
| **Group Levels of Organization** | |
| 1. Inability to engage in D-MT in the presence of others | |
| 2. Difficulty in sharing a movement session with others | |
| 3. Preoccupation with competition | |
| 4. Difficulty in involving self in short-term tasks | |
| 5. Difficulty in adopting group roles | |
| 6. Exhibitionistic, demands attention | |
| 7. Wants to excessively lead the group | |
| 8. Refuses to lead the group | |
| 9. Lack of minimal tolerance for closeness | |
| 10. Fear of dissolution of identity in a group | |
| 11. Self-referencing interferes with meeting others needs | |
| **Rites of Passage Levels of Organization** | |
| 1. Repressed fear from the birth trauma | |
| 2. Lack of basic trust in dyadic movement interactions | |
| 3. Difficulty in initiating any movement activities | |
| 4. Love-hate ambivalence with individuals of the opposite sex | |
| 5. Lack of sense of identity | |
| 6. Child-like or immature movement repertoire | |
| 7. Difficulty in commitment (vertical shape) | |
| 8. Lack of access to creative process | |
| 9. Sense of despair (flaccid, limp) | |

| | |
|---|---|
| 10. Sense of alientation and separateness (hollow and narrow and shortened shape flow) | |
| 11. Denial of anger concerning one's mortality | |
| 12. Difficulty in relating to the transpersonal | |
| 13. Lack of relationship to the soul | |
| Tactile Perceptual Levels of Organization | |
| 1. Excess amount of free flow | |
| 2. Lack of adaptive response to tactile stimulation | |
| 3. Tactile defensiveness | |
| 4. Seeks touch, clings | |
| 5. Difficulty in differentiating tactile stimulation | |
| 6. Difficulty in discriminating between positive and negative stimulation | |
| 7. Difficulty in retaining and recalling tactile stimulation | |
| Kinesthetic Perceptual Levels of Organization | |
| 1. Difficulty in recognizing proprioceptive stimuli | |
| 2. Difficulty in recognizing vibratory stimuli | |
| 3. Difficulty in discriminating or localizing kinesthetic stimuli | |
| 4. Poor position sense | |
| 5. Difficulty in retaining and recalling kinesthetic stimuli | |
| Vestibular Perceptual Levels of Organization | |
| 1. Difficulty in sensing or reacting to vestibular stimuli | |
| 2. Continuous loss of balance | |
| 3. Difficulty in discriminating vibratory stimuli | |
| 4. Difficulty in retaining and recalling stimuli and/or the appropriate response | |

Cognitive Representation Levels of Organization

| | |
|---|---|
| 1. Difficulty in enactive cognition | |
| 2. Difficulty in iconic cognition | |
| 3. Difficulty in abstract cognition | |

Thought Process Levels of Organization

| | |
|---|---|
| 1. Predominance of primary process thought | |
| 2. Dominance of symbolic inadaptive ritualized movement | |
| 3. Inability to differentiate between primary and secondary process thought | |
| 4. Lack of access to the unconscious | |
| 5. Overriding personal unconscious material | |
| 6. Inability to experience the archetypal | |
| 7. Lack of sense of one's personal journey | |

Play-Work Levels of Organization

| | |
|---|---|
| 1. Body insufficiently conditioned | |
| 2. Difficulty in moving improvisationally | |
| 3. Inability to utilize play as a transitional space | |
| 4. Difficulty in creative problem solving | |

## OUTLINE FOR MOVEMENT PROFILE
## (Adapted from Kestenberg Profile)[1]

Penny Bernstein, Ph.D., DTR

I. General Information
   A. Name
   B. Age
   C. Sex
   D. Date
   E. Circumstances (time, environment) under which observations were made

II. Profile
   A. Body Attitude
      1. Body alignment and favored position
      2. Shape flow position
      3. Two-effort quality of movement left imprinted on the body
      4. Dynamics and shape of breathing
      5. Characteristic effort shape phrase
   B. Tension flow rhythms (apparatus for discharge of drives)
      1. Dominant rhythm (fixation)
      2. Ratios of rhythms to each other (oral: anal: urethral: inner genital: outer genital (phallic))
      3. Characteristic rhythm
      4. Pure to mix rhythm ratio (3:1 appropriate for adult)
      5. Note presence or absence of all rhythms in pure form needed before drive differentiation can occur
      6. Dominant mixed rhythm (indicative of sublimation)
      7. Libidinal: sadistic rhythm ratio (more libidinal than sadistic in mixed rhythms appropriate for adaptive behavior)
      8. Presence of localization of rhythmic drive needed for ego control and mediation

1. Judith Kestenberg and Mark Sossin, *The Role of Movement Patterns in Development 2*. (New York: Dance Notation Bureau Press, 1979.)

C. Pre-efforts (reflect modes of learning and defenses against drives)
   1. Dominant pre-efforts employed in learning
   2. Dominant pre-efforts employed for ego defense mechanisms
      a. spatial pre-efforts (motor apparatuses for defense mechanisms)
         i. avoidance
         ii. deflection
         iii. isolation (channeling)
         iv. intellectualization
         v. emotional insulation (channeling)
      b. weight pre-efforts (motor apparatuses for defense mechanisms)
         i. identification with aggressor
         ii. defensive stubborness
         iii. reaction formation
      c. time pre-efforts (motor apparatuses for defense mechanisms)
         i. counter-phobic behavior
         ii. escape
      d. pre-effort combinations (motor apparatuses for defense mechanisms)
         i. time and weight pre-efforts
            —denial
            —repression
         ii. space and weight pre-efforts
            —projection

D. Efforts (ego mediation of drives in service to adaptation to reality)
   1. Posture—gesture
      a. gestural efforts (capabilities)
      b. postural efforts (punitive super ego, adaptation addressed to forbidden or permissible adaptive actions)

2. Gain expense ratio: ratio of effort attributes (e.g., light, direct, etc.) to flow changes (i.e., free to bound or bound to free) (relates to level of affect differentiation and complexity)
    a. 2:1 (reflects affect that is highly differentiated, lacking in spontaneity)
    b. 1:6 (reflects child-like spontaneity with little or no sublimation)
3. Characteristic effort phrase
4. Relationship of indulging to fighting efforts

E. Shape flow (id apparatus for the transfer of libidinal and aggressive tension flow impulses from self to objects)
1. Relationship of growing to shrinking
    a. level of self-representation and self-esteem
    b. shape flow changes (relates to level of plasticity)
2. Appropriate presence of symmetrical shape flow (delineating responses to the environment)
3. Appropriate presence of unilateral assymmetrical shape flow (delineating capacity to respond to discrete stimuli of positive and noxious natures)

F. Directional shape (express modes of object-related learning and defenses against objects)
1. Dominant directional shape employed
2. Relationship to objects (delineating again which relationships are defended)

G. Shaping (ego apparatus for complex relationship with the environnent and objects)
1. Posture—gesture
    a. gestural shaping (relates to self-appraisal)
    b. postural shaping (relates to superego functioning)
        i. ego ideal
        ii. aspirations and denigration of self in relation to objects
2. Characteristic shape phrase

H. Interrelationships within psychic structures

1. Id (tension and shape flow)
    a. homogeneous matching (consonance)
        i. dominant libidinal rhythms with growing shape flow
        ii. doninant aggressive/sadistic rhythms with shrinking shape flow
    b. intra systemic id conflicts
        i. dominant libidinal rhythms with shrinking shape flow
        ii. dominant aggressive/sadistic rhythms with growing shape flow
2. Ego (pre-efforts, efforts, dimensional shape, and shaping)
    a. homogeneous matching (consonance)
        i. presence of corresponding pre-efforts to efforts (e.g., presence of similar proportions of channeling and directness to flexibility and indirectness)
        ii. efforts matching with shapes (e.g., lightness with rising)
    b. intra systemic ego conflicts
        i. clashes between proportions of pre-efforts and proportion of effort actions
        ii. clashes between proportions of directional shape and shaping
        iii. clashes between related pre-efforts to directional shape
        iv. clashes between related efforts and shaping (demonstrates split between coping with the environment (efforts) and relating to objects (shapes)
            a) presence of shaping, absence of corresponding efforts demonstrates object orientation without needed adaptive dynamics
            b) presence of efforts, absence of corresponding shaping demonstrates adaptation to reality without relationship to objects

3. Superego (postural (P) efforts, postural (p) shapes)
   a. homogeneous matching (consonance) corresponding (P) efforts to (P) shapes
   b. intra systemic superego conflicts (mismatching of (P) efforts to corresponding (P) shapes—E.g., presence of (P) efforts with absence of (P) shaping indicates a lack of ego ideal internalization and a need to seek outside approval.)

III. Inter Systemic Relationship

| *ID* | *EGO* | *SUPEREGO* |
|---|---|---|
| oral | space efforts/horizontal shape | (P) spatial efforts/(P) horizontal shape |
| anal | weight efforts/vertical shape | (P) weight efforts/(P) vertical shape |
| urethral | time efforts/sagittal shape | (P) time efforts/(P) sagittal shape |

1. Id—Ego (tension, shape flow—efforts, shapes)
   a. matching
      1. rhythms with efforts (demonstrates appropriate ego mediation of drives)
      2. shape flow with shapes (demonstrates appropriate mediation of drives into object world)
   b. mis-matching (conflicts)
      1. rhythms with efforts (Rhythm dominance indicates loss of ego control of impulses.)
      2. shape flow with shapes (Shape flow dominance indicates impulsive relationship to objects.)
2. Ego—Superego (efforts, shapes—(P) efforts, (P) shapes)
   a. matching
      1. efforts to (P) efforts (indicates adaptation to reality syntonic with judging punitive superego—E.g., relationship of gestural indirectness corresponds to (P) indirectness.)
      2. shapes to (P) shapes (indicates object relationships consonant with ego ideal)

b. mis-matching (conflicts)
    1. efforts to (P) efforts (indicates how the individual adapts to reality is not in agreement with judgmental super ego, e.g., dominance of strength and quickness to (P) lightness and sustainment)
    2. shapes to (P) shapes (indicates relationship to objects is not syntonic with ego ideal)

IV. Conclusion
  A. Summary
  B. Recommendations
    1. appropriate treatment modality
    2. treatment goals
      a. long-term
      b. specific short-term
  C. Prognosis

# BIBLIOGRAPHY

## Books


Allport, J. W., and Vernon, P. E. *Studies in Expressive Movement.* New York: The Macmillan Company, 1933.

*American Journal of Dance Therapy.* Columbia:ADTA Publications, vols. 1–3, 1978–1980.

Arnheim, Rudolf. *Toward a Psychology of Art.* Los Angeles: University of California Press, 1966.

Assagioli, Roberto, Ed. *Synthesis: The Realization of the Self.* Redwood City: The Synthesis Press, vols. 1–2, 3–4, 1976, 1977.

Bartenieff, Irmgard, and Davis, Martha Ann. *Effort-Shape Analysis of Movement: The Unity of Expression and Function.* New York: Albert Einstein College of Medicine, 1963.

Beard, Ruth. *An Outline of Piaget's Developmental Psychology for Students and Teachers.* New York: Basic Books, Inc., 1969.

Bernstein, Penny, Ed. *Eight Theoretical Approaches in Dance-Movement Therapy.* Dubuque:Kendall/Hunt Publishing Company, 1979.

Birdwhistle, Ray. *Introduction to Kinesics.* Louisville: University of Louisville, 1967.

———. *Kinesics and Context.* Philadelphia: University of Pennsylvania, 1970.

Butter, Charles. *Neuropsychology: The Study of Brain and Behavior.* Belmont, Brooks/Cole Publishing Co., 1968.

Campbell, Joseph. *Hero with a Thousand Faces.* New York: World Pub. Co., 1970.

———. *Myths to Live By.* New York: Viking Press, 1972.

Castillejo, Irene Claremont de. *Knowing Woman.* New York: Harper and Row Pub., 1973.

Chaiklin, Harris. *Marian Chace:Her Papers.* Columbia: ADTA Publications, 1975.

Christiansen, Bjorn. *Thus Speaks the Body.* New York: Arno Press, 1972.

Cirlot, J. E. A *Dictionary of Symbols.* New York: Philosophical Library, 1978.

Cumming, John, and Cumming, Elaine. *Ego and Milieu.* New York: Atherlon Press, 1966.

Dell, Cecily. *A Primer for Movement Description.* New York: Dance Notation Bureau, 1970.

Deutsch, Felix. *On the Mysterious Leap from the Mind to the Body.* New York: International Universities Press, 1973.

*Diagnostic and Statistical Manual of Mental Disorders: DSM III.* Washington, D.C.:American Psychiatric Assoc., 1980.

Doubler, Margaret H. *Dance: A Creative Art Experience.* Madison: The University of Wisconsin Press, 1968.

Dunbar, Flanders. *Emotions and Bodily Changes.* New York: Columbia University Press, 1954.

Erikson, Erik. *Childhood and Society.* New York: W. W. Norton and Co., 1963.

Evan, Blanche. *The Child's World: Its Relation to Dance Pedagogy.* New York: Dance Therapy Center, 1948.

Evans-Wentz, W.Y., ed. *The Tibetan Book of the Dead.* London: Oxford University Press, 1960.

Fast, Julius. *Body Language.* New York: M. Evans & Co., 1970.

Federn, Paul. *Ego Psychology and the Psychoses.* New York: Basic Books, Inc., 1952.

Feldman, Sandor, M.D. *Mannerisms of Speech and Gestures.* New York: International Universities Press, 1971.

Fenichel, Otto. *The Psychoanalytic Theory of Neurosis.* New York: W. W. Norton, 1972.

Fiorentino, Mary. *Reflex Testing for Evaluating C.N.S. Development.* Springfield: Charles C. Thomas, 1965.

Fisher, Seymour. *Body Experience in Fantasy and Behavior.* New York: Appleton-Century-Crofts, 1970.

Ford, Donald, and Urban, Hugh. *Systems of Psychotherapy.* New York: John Wiley and Sons, Inc., 1967.

Freud, Anna. *Normality and Pathology in Childhood.* New York: International Universities Press, 1966.

———. *The Psychoanalytic Treatment of Children.* New York: Schocken Books, 1966.

Freud, Sigmund. *An Outline of Psychoanalysis.* New York: W. W. Norton & Co., 1949.

Gaston, E. Mayer, Ph.D. *Music in Therapy.* New York: Macmillan Company, 1968.

Gordon, Jesse, Ed. *Handbook of Clinical and Experimental Hypnosis.* New York: Macmillan Company, 1967.

Greenson, Ralph. *The Techniques and Practice of Psychoanalysis.* New York: International Universities Press, 1967.

Gunther, Bernard. *Sense Relaxation Below Your Mind.* New York: Macmillan Company, 1968.

Hall, Nor. *The Moon and The Virgin.* New York: Harper & Row, Pub., 1980.

Hanna, Judith Lynne. *To Dance Is Human.* Austin:University of Texas Press, 1979.

Harding, Esther. *Woman's Mysteries.* New York: Harper & Row, Pub., 1971.

Hartman, Heinz. *Ego Psychology and the Problem of Adaptation.* New York: International Universities Press, 1958.

Jung, C.G. *Man and His Symbols.* New York: Doubleday & Company, 1964.

———. *Memories Dreams and Reflections.* New York: Random House, 1961.

———. *On the Nature of the Psyche.* New York: Bollingen Foundation, 1960.

———. *The Practice of Psychotherapy.* New York: Pantheon Books, 1954.

Kephart, Newell. *The Slow Learner in the Classroom.* Columbus: Charles Merrill Books, 1960.

Kernberg, Otto. *Boarderline Conditions and Pathological Narcissism.* New York: Jason Aronson, Inc., 1979.

Kestenberg, Judith. *Children and Parents.* New York: Jason Aronson, Inc., 1975.

———, and Sossin, Mark. *The Role of Movement Patterns in Development II.* New York: Dance Notation Bureau, 1979.

King, Bruce. *Creative Dance Experience for Learning.* New York: Bruck King Studio, 1968.

Kohut, H. *The Analysis of the Self.* New York: International Universities Press, 1971.

Kubie, Lawrence. *Neurotic Distortion of the Creative Process.* Lawrence: University of Kansas Press, 1968.

Kris, Ernst. *Psychoanalytic Explorations in Art.* New York: Schocken Books, 1967.

Laban, Rudolf, and Lawrence, F. C. *Effort.* London: MacDonald and Evans, 1947.

———. *The Mastery of Movement.* London: MacDonald and Evans, 1960.

Lamb, Warren, and Watson, Elizabeth. *Body Code.* London: Routledge & Kegan Paul, 1979.

———, and Turner, David. *Management Behavior.* New York: International Universities Press, 1969.
———. *Posture and Gesture.* London: Gerald Duckworth & Co., Ltd., 1965.
Langer, Jonas; Mussen, Paul; and Covington, Martin, Eds. *Trends and Issues in Developmental Psychology.* New York: Holt, Rinehart & Winston, 1969.
Langer, Jonas. *Theories of Development.* New York: Holt, Rinehart and Winston, 1969.
Lifton, Walter. *Working with Groups.* New York: John Wiley and Sons, 1966.
Lomax, Alan. *Folk Song Style and Culture.* Washington, D.C.: Plimpton Press, 1968.
Lowen, Alexander. *The Betrayal of the Body.* New York: Macmillan Company, 1967.
———. *The Language of the Body.* New York: Collier Books, 1971.
Machover, Karen. *Personality Projection in the Drawing of the Human Figure.* Springfield: Charles C. Thomas, 1949.
Mahler, Margaret. *On Human Symbiosis and the Vicissitudes of Individuation.* New York: International Universities Press, 1968.
*Manual on Administration.* New York: American Occupational Therapy Assoc., 1965.
McGraw, Myrtle. *The Neuromuscular Maturation of the Human Infant.* New York: Hafner Company, 1966.
Meerloo, Joost A. M. *Creativity and Eternization: Essays on Creative Instinct.* New York: Humanities Press, 1968.
Middleman, Ruth. *The Non-Verbal Method in Working with Groups.* New York: Association Press, 1968.
Minuchen, Salvador. *Psychosomatic Families.* Cambridge: Harvard University Press, 1978.
Mosey, Anne. *Occupational Therapy: Theory and Practice.* Medford: Pothier Bros., 1968.
Muss, Rolf. *Theories of Adolescence.* New York: Ramdom House, 1969.
Mussen, Henry; Conger, John; and Kagan, Jerome. *Child Development and Personality.* New York: Harper and Row, 1963.
Neumann, Erich. *The Child.* New York: Harper & Row Pub., 1976.
North, Marian. *Personality Assessment Through Movement.* London: MacDonald and Evans, 1972.
Noyes, Arthur, and Kolb, Lawrence. *Modern Clinical Psychiatry.* Philadelphia: W. B. Saunders Company, 1964.
Pesso, Albert. *Experience in Action.* New York: New York University Press, 1973.
Piaget, Jean; Inhelder, Barbel; and Szeminska, Alina. *The Child's Conception of Geometry.* New York: Basic Books, Inc., 1960.
———. *The Origins of Intelligence in Children.* New York: W. W. Norton & Co., 1963.
Perls, Frederick, M.D., Ph.D.; Hefferline, Ralph, Ph.D.; Goodman, Paul, Ph.D. *Gestalt Therapy.* New York: Dell Publishing Company, 1951.
Preston, Valerie. *A Handbook for Modern Educational Dance.* London: MacDonald & Evans, 1963.
Ramsden, Pamela. *Top Team Planning.* New York: John Wiley and Sons, 1973.
Rosen, John. *Direct Analysis.* New York: Grune & Stratton, 1953.
Russell, Joan. *Creative Dance in the Primary School.* New York: Frederick Praeger, 1968.
Schilder, Paul. *Brain and Personality.* New York: International Universities Press, 1951.
———. *The Image and Appearance of the Human Body.* New York: John Wiley & Sons, Inc., 1964.

Schmais, Claire, and Orleans, Florette, Eds. *Seven Pilot Studies.* New York: Hunter College, 1977.

Schoop, Trudi. *Won't You Join the Dance.* Palo Alto: National Press Books, 1974.

Schutz, William. *Joy: Expanding Human Awareness.* New York: Grove Press, 1968.

Sechehaye, Marguerite. *Autobiography of a Schizophrenic Girl.* New York: Grune and Stratton, 1965.

Shorr, Joseph, et. al., Eds. *Imagery: Its many Dimensions and Applications.* New York: Plenum Press, 1980.

Sullivan, Harry Stack. *Clinical Studies in Psychiatry.* New York: W. W. Norton & Co., 1956.

Thass-Thienemann, Theodore. *Symbolic Behavior.* New York: Washington Square Press, Inc., 1968.

Turner, Victor. *The Ritual Process Structure and Anti-Structure.* Chicago: Aldine Publishing Co., 1969.

Urban, William. *The Draw a Person.* Los Angeles: Western Psychological Services, 1973.

Von Franz, Marie-Louise. *Alchemical Active Imagination.* Dallas: Spring Publications, Inc., 1979.

———. *Interpretation of Fairytales.* Dallas: Spring Publications, 1978.

Wallace, Anthony. *Culture and Personality.* New York: Random House, 1969.

Whiting, John, and Child, Irwin. *Child Training and Personality.* New Haven: Yale University Press, 1953.

———, ———, and Lambert, William. *Field Guide for a Study of Socialization.* New York: John Wiley and Sons, Inc., 1966.

Willard, Helen, and Spackman, Clare. *Occupational Therapy.* Philadelphia: J. D. Lippincott Company, 1963.

Winnicott, D. W, *Mother and Child.* New York: Basic Books, Inc., 1957.

———. *The Family and Individual Development.* London: Tavistock Pub., 1965.

———. *The Maturational Processes and the Facilitating Environment.* New York: International Universities Press, 1965.

Wolff, Werner. *The Expression of Personality.* New York: Harper and Bros., 1945.

Wolman, Benjamin, Ed. *Dictionary of Behavioral Science.* New York: Van Nostrand Reinhold Company, 1973.

Zinker, Joseph. *Creative Process in Gestalt Therapy.* New York: Vintage Books, 1977.


## Articles and Unpublished Manuscripts


Adler, Janet. "The Study of an Autistic Child," *American Dance Therapy Association Conference Proceedings,* October, 1968.

Bartenieff, Irmgard. "Effort Observation and Effort Assessment in Rehabilitation," Dance Notation Bureau Reprint, New York, 1962.

———; Davis, Martha; and Paulay, Forestine. "Four Adaptations of Effort Theory in Research and Teaching," Dance Notation Bureau Reprint, New York, 1968.

———. "Research in Anthropology: A Study of Dance Styles in Primitive Cultures," *CORD,* May, 1967

Bender, Lauretta, and Boas, Franziska. "Creative Dance in Therapy," *American Journal of Orthopsychiatry,* April 1941.

Benedict, Ruth. "Child Rearing in Eastern European Countries," *Personalities and Cultures,* Robert Hunt, Ed. New York: Natural History Press, 1967.

Bernstein, Penny, and Bernstein, Lawrence. "A Conceptualization of Group Dance-Movement Therapy as a Ritual Process," *American Dance Therapy Association Monograph III,* 1974.

Bernstein, Penny. "A Mythologic Quest: Jungian Movement Therapy with the Psychosomatic Client," *American Journal of Dance Therapy,* Spring, 1980.

———, and Cafarelli, Enzo. "An Electromyographical Validation of the Effort System of Notation," *American Dance Therapy Association Monograph II.,* 1973

———, and Hall, Leah. "Cross-Cultural Puberty Rituals and Jungian Dance Therapy," paper presented at First International Dance Therapy Assoc. Conference, Toronto, 1977.

———. "Dance-Movement Therapy" *Psychotherapy Handbook,* Richard Herink, Ed. New York: New American Library, 1980.

———, and Garson, Blaine. "Pilot Study in the Use of Tension Flow System of Movement Notation in an Ongoing Study of Infants as Risk for Schizophrenic Disorders," *Dance Therapy—Depth and Dimension,* Delores Plunk, Ed. ADTA, 1975.

———. "Range of Response as seen Through a Developmental Progression," *What is Dance Therapy Really?,* Govine and Smallwood, Eds. ADTA, 1973.

———. "Tension Flow Rhythms As a Developmental Diagnostic Tool Within the Theory of the Recapitulation of Ontogeny," *Dance Therapy —Depth and Dimension,* Delores Plunk, ED. ADTA, 1975.

———. "The Union of the Gestalt Concept of Experiment and Jungian Active Imagination," *The Gestalt Journal,* Fall, 1980.

Chace, M. "A Psychological Study as Applied to Dance," Presented at the American Psychological Association Meetings, New York, September, 1957.

———. "Dance as an Adjunctive Therapy with Hospitalized Mental Patients," *Bulletin of the Menninger Clinic,* XVIX, November 1953, pp. 219–25.

———. "Dance as Communication: Its Use in Growth or Treatment Situations." (Unpublished manuscript).

———. "Measurable and Intangible Aspects of Dance Sessions," *Music Therapy,* VII 1957, pp. 151–156.

———. "Movement Communication with Children," *American Dance Therapy Association Conference Proceedings,* October, 1968.

———. "The Role of the Psychiatric Nurse in Dance Sessions," *St. Mary's Newsletter,* VIII, October, 1960, p. 8.

———. "Stimulation of Creative Forms in Patient Productions." Presented at the Southeastern Chapter of the National Association for Music Therapy, Columbia, South Carolina, March 7, 1958.

———. "Technique for the Use of Dance as a Group Therapy," *Music Therapy,* III (1954), pp. 62–67.

———. "Use of Dance Action in Group Setting." Presented at the American Psychiatric Association Meeting, Los Angeles, California, May, 1943.

Chaiklin, Harris. "Research and the Development of a Profession," *American Dance Therapy Association Conference Proceedings,* October, 1968.

Condon, W. S. "Kinesic Research and Dance Therapy," *American Dance Therapy Association Conference Proceedings,* October, 1968.

Dratman, Mitchell L. "Reorganization of Psychic Structures in Autism: A Study Using Body Movement Therapy," *American Dance Therapy Association Conference Proceedings,* October, 1967.

Duffy, E. "The Measurement of Muscular Tension as a Technique for the Study of Emotional Tendencies," *American Journal of Psychology,* XLIV, 1932, pp. 146–162.

Dyrud, Jack; Chace, Marian; and Erdman, Jean. "The Meaning of Movement as Human Expression and as an Artistic Communication," *American Dance Therapy Association Conference Proceedings,* October, 1968.

Ferman, John, and Vargue, James. "Dimensions of Growth," *Synthesis,* vol. 3–4, 1977.

Grindlach, Ralph. "Movement Research," *CORD,* May 26, 1961, Introduction.

Hanna, Judith. "Dance Field Research: Some Whys and African Wherefores," *CORD,* May 1967.

Harrington, Charles. "Sexual Differentiation in Socialization and Some Male Genital Mutilations," *American Anthropologist,* LXX, October, 1968.

Howe, Louisa. "Notes on a Freudian Formulation of Psychomotor Therapy," Unpublished manuscript.

James, William T. "A Study of the Expression of Bodily Posture," *The Journal of Genetic Psychology,* VII, 1932, pp. 405–37.

Kalish, Beth. "Body Movement Therapy for Autistic Children," *American Dance Therapy Association Conference Proceedings,* October, 1968.

Kestenberg, Judith. "Childhood and Adult Pathology," *Journal of Hillside Hospital,* XVII, April-July, 1968.

———. "Notes on Parenthood as a Developmental Phase," paper presented at the American Psychoanalytic Assoc., Denver, 1974.

———. "Prevention, Infant Therapy, and the Treatment of Adults," reprint available at Sands Point Child Development Center, 1978.

———. "Rhythm and Organization in Obsessive-Compulsive Development," *The International Journal of Psycho-Analysis,* XLVII, 1966, pp. 151–159.

———. "The Role of Movement Patterns in Development: I. Rhythms of Movement," *Psychoanalytic Quarterly,* XXXIV, 1965, pp. 1–36.

———. "The Role of Movement Patterns in Development: II," *Psychoanalytic Quarterly,* XXXIV, 1965, pp. 517–562.

———. "The Role of Movement Patterns in Development: III. The Control of Shape," *Psychoanalytic Quarterly,* XXXVI, 1967, pp. 359–409.

———. "Self-Environment and Objects as Seen Through the Study of Movement Patterns," Unprinted manuscript, 1969.

———. "Suggestions for Diagnostic and Therapeutic Procedures in Movement Therapy," *American Dance Therapy Association Conference Proceedings,* October, 1967.

Krout, Maurice, "A Preliminary Note on Some Obscure Symbolic Muscular Responses of Diagnostic Value in the Study of Normal Subjects," *American Journal of Psychiatry,* II, 1931–2. pp. 29–71.

La Barre, Weston. "The Cultural Basis of Emotions and Gestures," *Journal of Personality,* XVI, 1947, pp. 48–68.

Lippman, Paul. "Is There Life Before Death? Schizophrenia, Normality and Other Human Disasters" *American Dance Therapy Association Conference Proceedings,* October, 1968.

Lowen, Alexander. "Breathing, Movement, and Feeling," Lecture reprint, 1965.

———. "The Rhythm of Life," Lecture reprint, 1966.

———. "Sex and Personality," Lecture reprint, 1962.

———. "Thinking and Feeling," Lecture reprint, 1967.

Mosey, Anne. "Treatment of Pathological Distortion of Body Image," *The American Journal of Occupational Therapy,* XXIII, September-October, 1969.

Pesso, Albert. "Workshop on Psychomotor Therapy," *American Dance Therapy Association Conference Proceedings,* October, 1968.

Rubin, Judith; Irwin, Eleanor; and Bernstein, Penny. "Play, Parenting, and the Arts, "*Therapeutic Process: Movement as Integration,* Penny Bernstein, Ed., Columbia: ADTA, 1975.

Salome-Finkelstein. "An Experimental Psychological Study of the Kinetic Pattern in Schizophrenia," *Psychiatria Neurologia Neurochirurgia,* LXVII, 1964, pp. 182–186.

Schmals, Claire, and White, Elissa. "Movement Analysis for Dance Therapists," *American Dance Therapy Association Conference Proceedings,* 1969.

Vaughn, Frances, and Walsh, Roger. "Beyond the Ego: Toward Transpersonal Models of the Person and Psychology," *Journal of Humanistic Psychology,* vol. 20, no. 1, 1980.

Zwerling, Israel. "The Creative Arts Therapies as 'Real Therapies,' " *Hospital and Community Psychiatry,* Dec., 1979.

———. "The Creative Arts Therapies: Struggling for Recognition," *Hospital and Community Psychiatry,* Dec., 1979.

## Films

Adler, Janet. *Looking for Me.* Produced by Maurice Falk Medical Fund, Pittsburgh, 1970.

Bernstein, Penny. *To Move Is to Be Alive: A Developmental Approach in Dance Movement Therapy.* Produced by Pittsburgh Child Guidance Center and Maurice Falk Medical Fund, Pittsburgh, 1973.

Kalish, Beth. *Film of Dance Therapy with an Autistic Child.* Philadelphia.

# INDEX